国家心血管病中心
中国医学科学院阜外医院
心血管外科年度报告2023

主 编 胡盛寿

National Center For Cardiovascular Diseases

Fuwai Hospital, Chinese Academy of Medical Sciences,
Peking Union Medical College

CARDIOVASCULAR SURGERY

OUTCOMES 2023

中国协和医科大学出版社
北 京

图书在版编目（CIP）数据

国家心血管病中心中国医学科学院阜外医院心血管外科年度报告. 2023 / 胡盛寿主编. -- 北京：中国协和医科大学出版社, 2024.8.-- ISBN 978-7-5679-2451-2

Ⅰ. R654

中国国家版本馆CIP数据核字第2024SL0159号

主　　编　胡盛寿

责任编辑　李元君　胡安霞

封面设计　邱晓俐

责任校对　张　麓

责任印制　黄艳霞

出版发行　**中国协和医科大学出版社**
（北京市东城区东单三条9号　邮编100730　电话010-65260431）

网　　址　www.pumcp.com

印　　刷　小森印刷（北京）有限公司

开　　本　889mm×1194mm　　1/16

印　　张　5.5

字　　数　150千字

版　　次　2024年8月第1版

印　　次　2024年8月第1次印刷

定　　价　120.00元

（版权所有，侵权必究，如有印装质量问题，由本社发行部调换）

编者名单

主　编　胡盛寿

副主编　郑　哲　赵　韡　袁　昕

编　者　袁　靖　陈　凯　储　庆　高仕君

　　　　饶辰飞　罗明尧　马　凯　王玉鑫

　　　　陈蔚南　王海彬　武新华

院长寄语
President's address

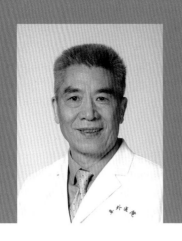

尊敬的广大同仁及患者朋友们，大家好！

很高兴2023年阜外医院心血管外科年度报告与大家见面。过去一年是疫情结束后的第一年，我院不仅常见外科疾病就诊量大幅攀升，而且急危重症患者就诊比例也明显增加。阜外医院心血管外科同仁本着"患者至上"的原则，为广大患者提供了高品质的医疗服务，在业内发挥了重要的龙头引领作用。

现代科技的飞速发展给健康产业带来了深刻变革，新体系、新趋势、新效能、新动力、新文化不断冲击着旧有公立医院运营模式。以高质量发展为目标，建立以大数据为基础的医院管理信息化、智能化、网络化、自动化体系至关重要。

如何科学有效地进行医疗质控？如何整合院内外一体化服务？如何加强医疗文书书写的科学性、准确性、及时性？如何通过电子病历系统改进医生行为、使共识和指南成为医生临床实践的自觉行为？如何利用大数据模型和智能模拟器加强对年轻医生的培养？如何对各级医生的临床实践能力进行考核，以促进"良医"的成长？

一系列重大课题对现有医院管理体系发起了挑战、也为高水平医院的进一步发展提供了机遇。在过去的一年中，我们在创造临床工作质与量双重新高的同时，依托"智慧化"信息平台，对上述重大医院管理问题进行了深入探索。今年的年报将尝试对去年工作做更全面的呈现和总结，以供心血管外科同道参考、批评、指正。

为心血管疾病患者提供优质而有温度的服务、引领我国心血管外科发展是阜外全体外科同仁永恒不变的追求！

国家心血管病中心主任

中国医学科学院阜外医院院长

中国工程院院士

2024年6月

目 录
Table of Contents

一、概况   1

二、冠状动脉粥样硬化性心脏病外科治疗   13

三、心脏瓣膜病与房颤外科治疗   21

四、主动脉及外周血管疾病外科治疗   31

五、先天性心脏病外科治疗   40

六、结构性心脏病外科治疗   51

七、晚期心脏病外科治疗   60

八、术后患者的全程康复和生活方式医学的推广   67

九、信息化、智能化助力医院高质量发展   77

一、概况
Overview

▶ 概述

2023年，门诊量、住院人数和手术量迎来了明显增长。医院心血管外科手术共计18 874例。尽管工作强度显著增大，医疗质量仍维持高水平不变。术后30日死亡率为0.4%，已连续15年低于1%，在世界各大心脏中心居于领先水平（图1-1）。

In 2023，a total of 18874 cardiovascular surgeries were performed，with a 30-day postoperative mortality rate of 0.4%. The rate has been kept below 1% for 15 consecutive years，which is at a leading level among big cardiac centers around the world（Figure 1-1）.

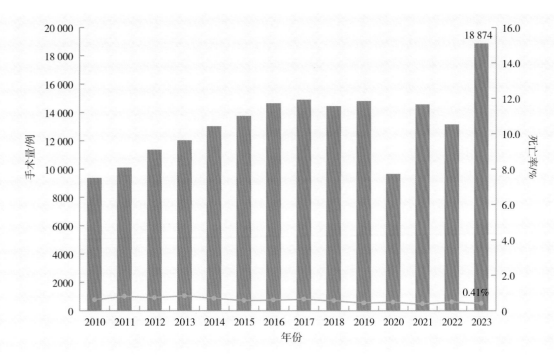

图1-1　2010—2023年心血管外科手术量及术后30日死亡率
Figure1-1　Volume and 30-day mortality, 2010—2023

医院收治患者的病因学分类基本反映了我国心血管外科疾病治疗谱。先天性心脏病和风湿性瓣膜病呈总体下降趋势，而冠状动脉粥样硬化性心脏病、退行性瓣膜病、主动脉外科手术等呈总体增加趋势（图1-2）。

The etiology characteristics of the patients in Fuwai Hospital reflects the profile of cardiovascular surgical diseases in China. Congenital heart diseases and rhematic valvular diseases are decreasing, while surgeries for coronary artery deases, degenerative valvular diseases and aortic diseases are increasing（Figure 1-2）.

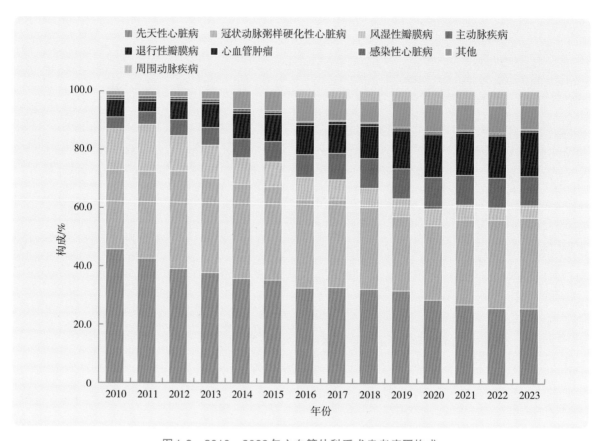

图1-2　2010—2023年心血管外科手术患者病因构成

Figure 1-2　Classification of etiology, 2010—2023

不同种类的心血管外科手术术后30日死亡率已连续多年均低于1%（图1-3），这体现了阜外医院在心血管外科手术的规范化管理、整体医疗质量的控制和疾病的综合救治水平均已达到世界先进水平。

The 30-day mortalities of cardiovascular surgeries is less than 1% for 15 years，which attribute to the standardized management of cardiovascular surgical procedures，the overall control of medical quality，and the comprehensive treatment for cardiovascular diseases in Fuwai hospital that have reached advanced world level（Figure 1-3）.

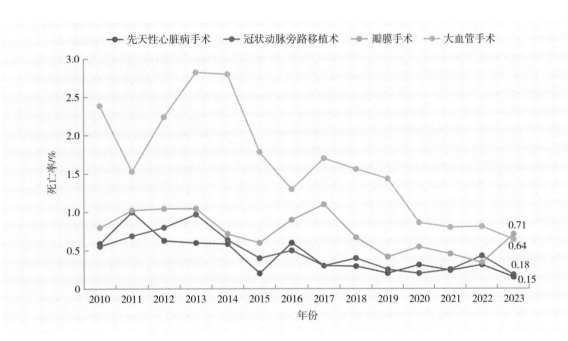

图1-3　2010—2023年心血管外科分术种手术死亡率

Figure 1-3　Mortality rates of cardiovascular surgeries, 2010—2023

在外科、重症医学科、临床检验科、影像科、心脏康复中心等多学科共同努力和紧密配合下，2023年，外科全术种的平均术后住院天数下降至8天以内，较去年进一步降低（图1-4）。

With a close cooperation of multiple department of cardiovascular surgery，intensive care unite，clinical laboratory，imaging，and cardiac rehabilitation center，the postoperative hospital stay of all surgical procedures in our hospital remains within 8 days，which is much shorter than last year（Figure 1-4）.

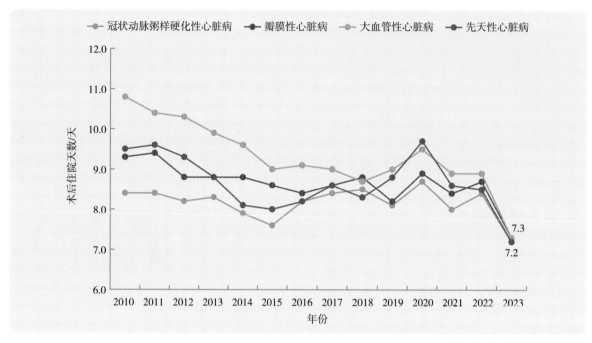

图1-4 2010—2023年心血管外科分术种术后住院天数
Figure 1-4 Postoperative length of stay, 2010—2023

自始至终，医院严格把控用血指征，不断提升围手术期血液保护和管理水平，改变了过去心血管外科"用血大户"的形象（图1-5、图1-6）。

From beginning，Fuwai strictly controlled the indications for blood use，continuously improved the level of perioperative blood protection and management，and changed the image of a "blood user" in cardiovascular surgery in the past（Figure 1-5，Figure 1-6）.

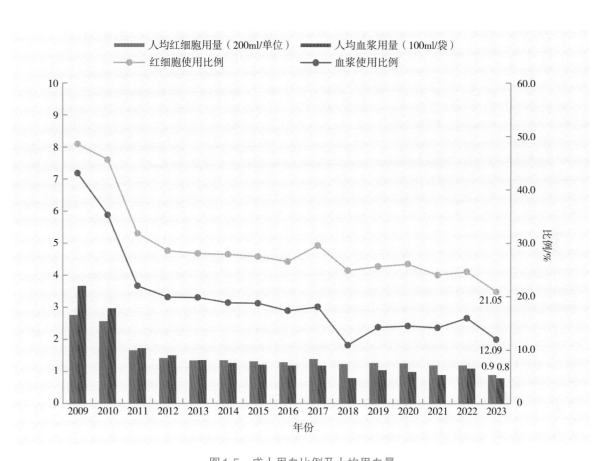

图1-5　成人用血比例及人均用血量

Figure 1-5　Blood use and average blood use in adult cardiac surgery

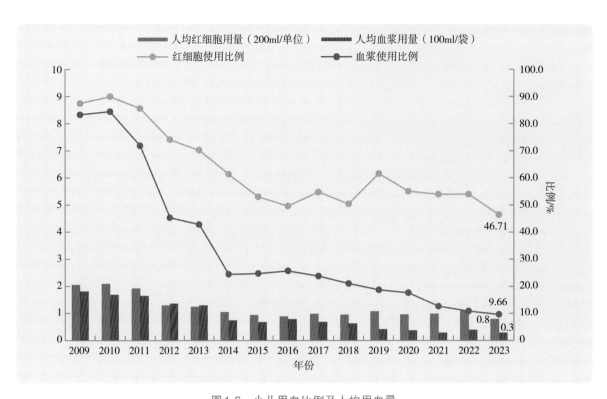

图1-6　小儿用血比例及人均用血量

Figure 1-6　Blood use and average blood use in pediatric cardiac surgery

2023年，急诊心血管手术量已超过2019年水平，急诊心血管手术死亡率较2022年有了进一步降低（图1-7）。

By the year 2023, the volume of emergency surgeries has greater than in 2019. The mortality of emergency surgeries is decreased compared to 2022（Figure 1-7）.

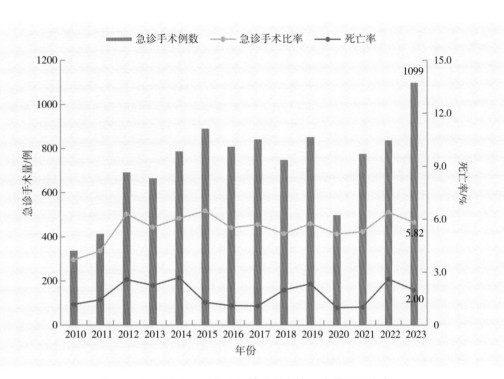

图1-7　2010—2023年心血管外科急诊手术量及死亡率

Figure 1-7　Volume of emergency surgery and the mortality rate, 2010-2023

60岁以上的老年人在总手术人群中占比逐年增加（图1-8），这是我国人口老龄化的体现，也说明心血管外科手术的风险在逐年提高。

The rate of patient aged 60 and above increases annually（Figure 1-8），which reflects the aging of the population in China. Therefore, the risk of cardiovascular surgery is increasing.

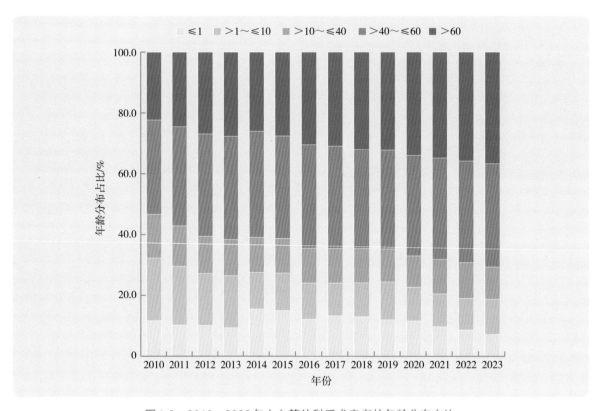

图1-8　2010—2023年心血管外科手术患者的年龄分布占比

Figure1-8　Age distribution of patients, 2010—2023

▶ 分中心与技术协作中心

推动国家级优质医疗资源扩容下沉，体现"国家队"情怀担当（图1-9～图1-10）。

Promote the expansion and sinking of high-quality medical resources at the national level, reflecting the spirit and responsibility of the "national team"（Figure 1-9 ~ Figure 1-10）.

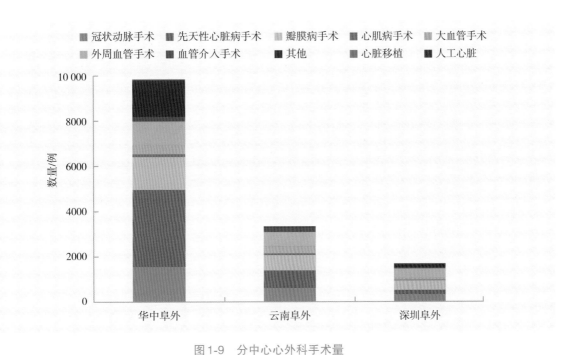

图1-9　分中心心外科手术量

Figure 1-9　Volume of cardiovascular surgery in branch hospitals of Fuwai.

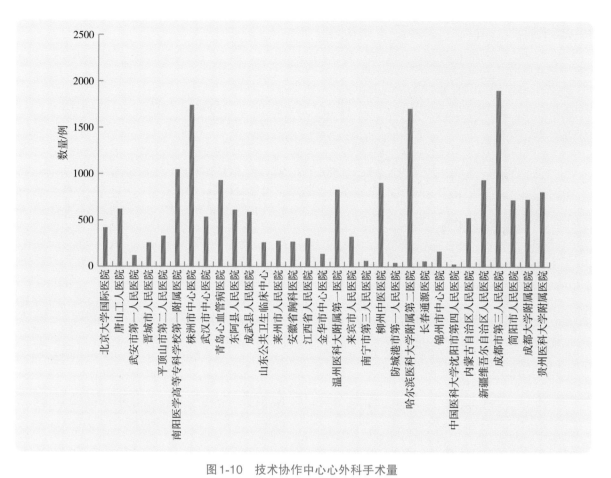

图1-10 技术协作中心心外科手术量

Figure 1-10 Volume of cardiovascular surgery in technical collaborating centers

▶ 学术会议（图1-11 ~ 图1-14）

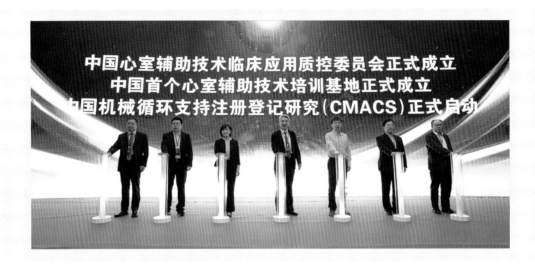

图1-11　成人心外科中心主办15场学术会议，举办6期技术培训班涵盖了冠脉、瓣膜、心脏移植、左心室辅助等多项技术交流

Figure 1-11　The Adult Cardiac Surgery Center hosted 15 academic conferences and six technical training courses, including coronary artery surgery, valvular surgery, heart transplantation and left ventricular assist device

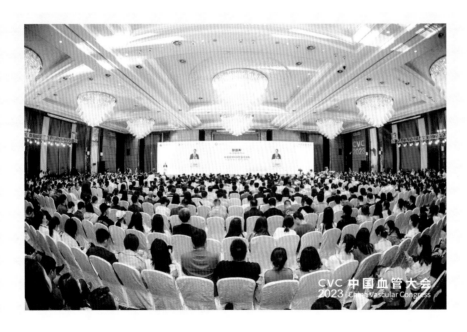

图1-12　血管外科中心主办中国血管大会和主动脉病变研讨会等四场国际、国内学术会议

Figure 1-12　The Vascular Surgery Center hosted four international and domestic academic conferences, including the China Vascular Conference and the Aortic Disease Symposium

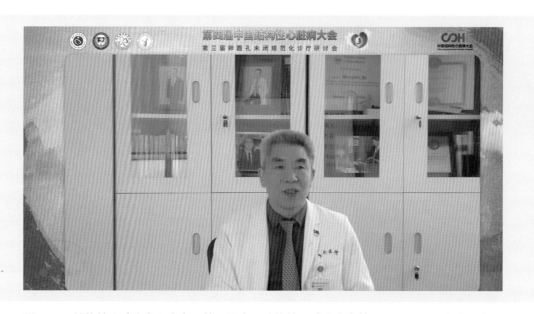

图1-13　结构性心脏病中心主办了第四届中国结构性心脏病大会等四场国际、国内学术会议

Figure 1-13　The Structural Heart Disease Center hosted four international and domestic academic conferences, including the 4th China Structural Heart Disease Conference

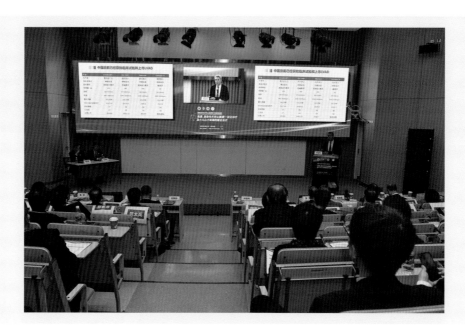

图1-14　小儿心外科中心成功举办复杂先天性心脏病研讨会和CHC先天性心脏病论坛

Figure 1-14　The Pediatric Cardiac Surgery Center held the Complex Congenital Heart Disease Seminar and the CHC Congenital Heart Disease Forum

二、冠状动脉粥样硬化性心脏病外科治疗
Coronary artery diseases

▶ **概述**

2023年，冠状动脉旁路移植术手术量较往年有显著增长，30日死亡率保持低水平。共完成冠状动脉旁路移植术6680例，其中单纯冠状动脉旁路移植术（coronary artery bypass grafting，CABG）4962例，30日死亡率已连续10年低于0.5%（图2-1）。

In 2023，the volume of CABG sets a new record and the 30-day mortality remains at very low level. 6680 patients underwent isolated or combined CABG at Fuwai Hospital, with 4962 cases being isolated CABG. The 30-day mortality has remained stable over the past 10 years at a level of less than 0.5%（Figure 2-1）.

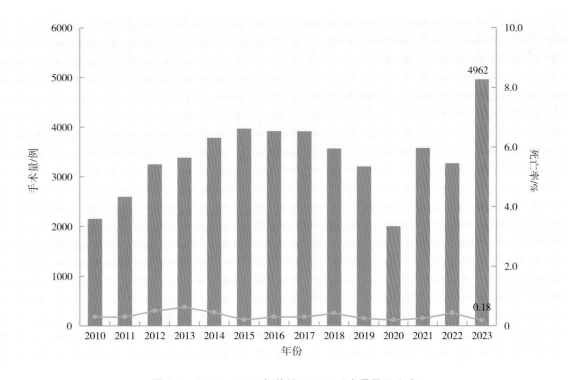

图 2-1　2010—2023 年单纯 CABG 手术量及死亡率

Figure2-1　Volume and mortality of isolated coronary artery bypass grafting, 2010—2023

患者的康复依赖于高水平的手术技术、围手术期管理监护水平和康复管理水平。2023年，单纯CABG手术的平均术后住院天数为7.01天，较前均有所降低（图2-2）。

The best recovery depends on outstanding surgical technique, post-operative care and cardiac rehabilitation. The length of stay for isolated CABG is 7.0 days in 2023（Figure 2-2）.

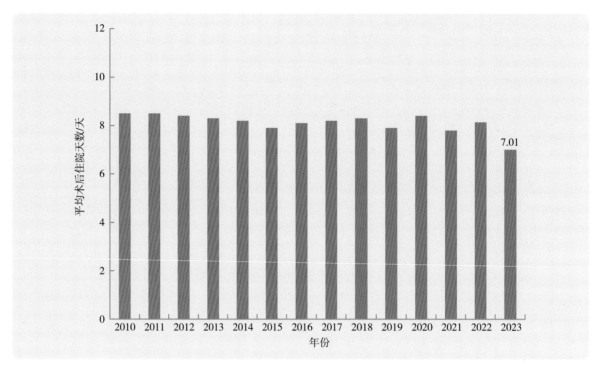

图2-2　2010—2023年单纯CABG手术患者平均术后住院天数

Figure2-2　Post-operative length of stoy of CABG, 2010—2023

▶ **典型病例**

急性心肌梗死心脏破裂患者抢救性手术治疗（图2-3）。

Emergency surgery for patients with acute myocardial infarction and cardiac rupture （Figure2-3）.

- 患者，男，77岁。急性心肌梗死，就诊于我院急诊，UCG提示大量心包积液，左心室前壁可见破口，EF 32%，考虑心脏破裂。来院时休克状态。
- 医院绿色通道，就诊2小时内快速完善检查并紧急手术。术中探查见大量心包积液、心包内大量血栓、左心室前壁心外膜破口。予以心脏破口及水肿心肌缝合，并行前降支、后降支搭桥。
- 患者术后带IABP返回监护室，后逐渐撤除辅助装置，顺利恢复出院。
- 本例患者病情危重，确诊后立刻动员我院绿色通道，快速完成术前准备，并顺利完成抢救手术，体现出了我院急重症心血管疾病的多学科诊治水平。
- A 77 year old male in shock with acute myocardial infarction was admitted to the emergency department. UCG showed a large amount of pericardial effusion, with a visible rupture in the left ventricular anterior wall. The LVEF was 32%.
- The hospital's green channel allows for quick and comprehensive examination and emergency surgery within 2 hours of diagnosis. During the surgery the rupture was fixed, and bypass grafting was performed. The patient returned to the ICU with IABP after surgery. The patient recovered and discharged finally.
- The successful rescue of the patient represented the high-level of multidisciplinary diagnosis and treatment for acute and severe cardiovascular diseases in Fuwai hospital.

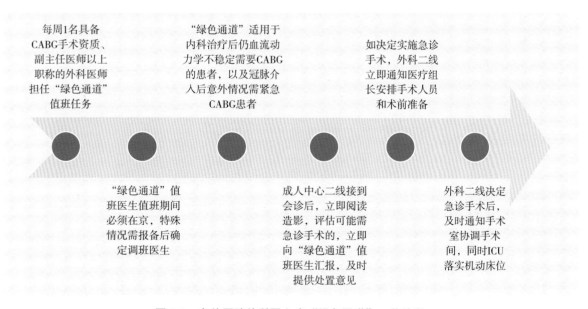

图2-3　阜外医院外科冠心病"绿色通道"工作流程

Figure 2-3　The "Green Channel" workflow for coronary artery surgery in Fuwai hospital

▶ 强化关键指标

    阜外医院动脉桥的使用率维持在95%以上。我们根据患者个体情况优化治疗策略，常规开展双侧乳内动脉、桡动脉和全动脉化等技术，旨在为不同患者提供高质量、个性化的血运重建策略（图2-4）。

    The use of left internal thoracic artery is over 95% for years at Fuwai hospital. The surgical teams intend to provide individualized optimal revascularization strategies for patients. Multiple approaches，such as bilateral internal thoracic artery，radial artery，and total arterial grafts，are also routinely performed in Fuwai hospital（Figure 2-4）.

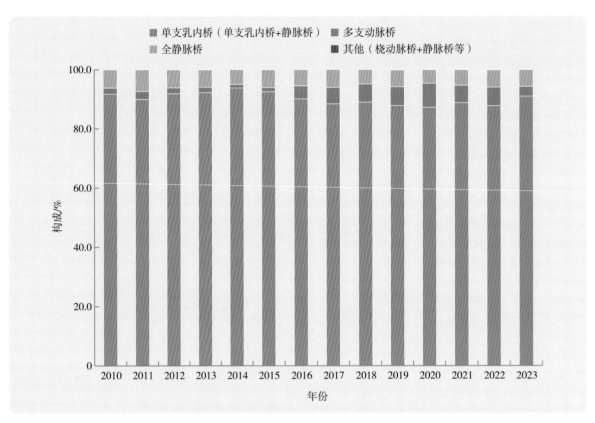

图2-4　2010—2023年单纯CABG移植物构成

Figure2-4　Usage of bypass conduits in CABG, 2010—2023

▶ 学术聚焦

No-touch技术获取静脉用于冠状动脉旁路移植——3年随访结果（图2-5）。

Graft Patency between No-Touch Vein Harvesting Technique and Conventional Approach in Coronary Artery Bypass Graft Surgery（PATENCY）（Figure2-5）.

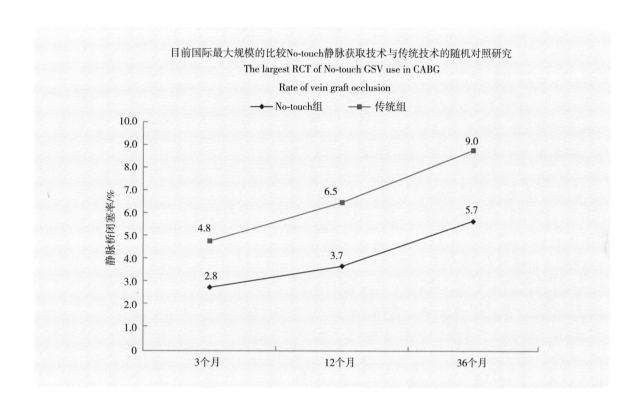

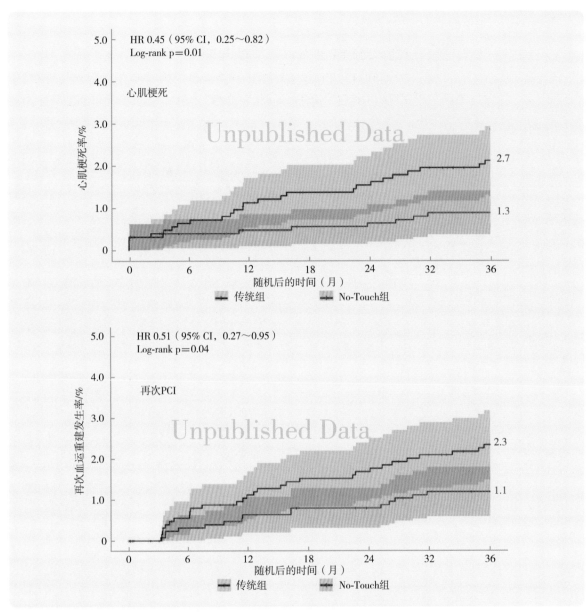

图2-5 No-touch技术获取静脉用于冠状动脉旁路移植——3年随访结果

Figure 2-5 Three-year results of No-touch technique for harvesting veins in coronary artery bypass grafting

注：No-touch技术显著降低CABG术后3年静脉桥闭塞率、心肌梗死、再次血运重建发生率。

No-touch technology significantly reduces the incidence of GSV occlusion，myocardial infarction, and revascularization after CABG surgery for 3 years.

基于QFR选择桡动脉桥的靶血管有重要意义（图2-6）。

Quantitative flow ratio（QFR）vs. Angiographic degree of stenosis（DS）（Figure2-6）.

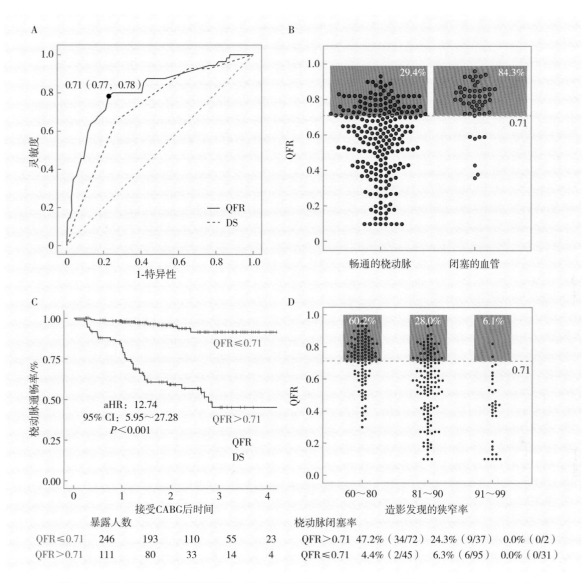

图2-6　相比于造影狭窄程度评估，靶血管QFR可以更好预测桡动脉闭塞率（界值为0.71）

Figure 2-6　QFR outperforms degree of stenosis in predicting RA anastomosis occlusion with the best cutoff value of 0.71

注：A、B.预测桡动脉桥闭塞——QFR优于DS。Predicting RA ocdusion；C、D.桡动脉通畅率QFR≤0.71远高于QFR＞0.71时。QFR outperforms DS；CUT off value of 0.71。

CABG术后抗血小板用药策略——双抗*vs*降阶梯

冠状动脉旁路移植术后降阶梯抗血小板治疗有效性、安全性研究（TOP-CABG Trial）（图2-7）。

The timing of platelet inhibition after coronary artery bypass grafting（TOP-CABG）（Figure2-7）.

● 多中心、随机、双盲、随机对照临床试验。

● 研究中心16所，受试者2300例。

Multicentre，randomised，double-blind，controlled trial

16 centers，2300 subjects

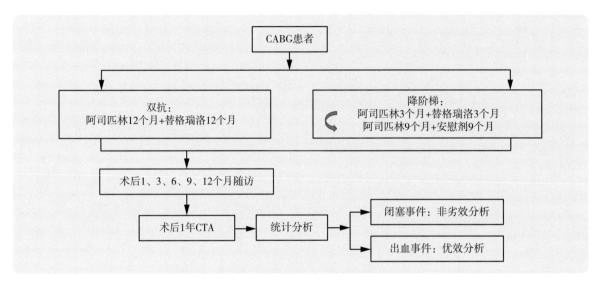

图2-7　TOP-CABG 研究流程图

Figure 2-7　The workflow of the TOP-CABG Trial

三、心脏瓣膜病与房颤外科治疗
Valvular heart diseases and surgical therapy of atrial fibrillation

► **概述**

    阜外医院是我国最大的瓣膜外科中心。2023年，我院共完成心脏瓣膜手术6479例，术后30日死亡率仅为0.5%（图3-1）。

    Fuwai Hospital is the largest cardiac valve surgery center in China. In 2023，6479 patients received valvular operation in Fuwai hospital with a 30-day mortality of 0.5%（Figure 3-1）.

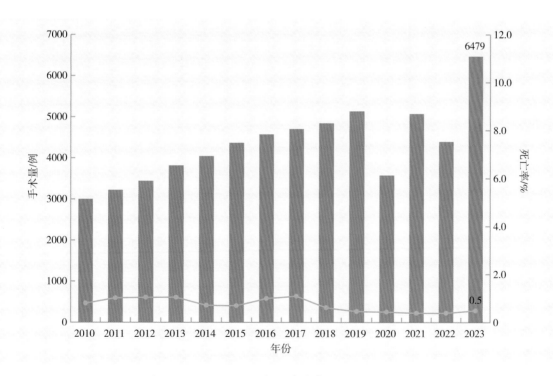

图3-1 2010—2023年心脏瓣膜手术量及死亡率

Figure3-1 Volume and mortality of cardiac valve surgery, 2010—2023

瓣膜外科疾病病因占比变化显著，退行性变和先天性病因占比已超过风湿性病变，成为目前瓣膜病的主要病因，这也对瓣膜外科的治疗技术提出了新的要求（图3-2）。

　　The etiology of valvular heart diseases changes significantly，Currently，degenerative valve disease and congenital valve disease has surpassed rheumatic valve disease，and became the major causes，which requested modern surgical techniques（Figure 3-2）.

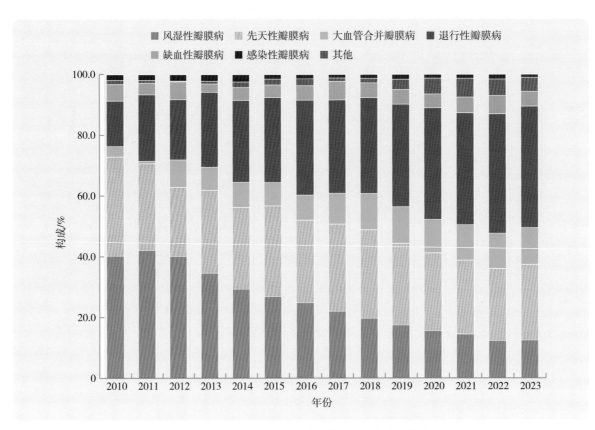

图3-2　2010—2023年心脏瓣膜手术患者病因构成

Figure 3-2　Etiology of valvular heart diseases

瓣膜手术的术后平均住院天数是重要的医疗质量评价指标。阜外医院心脏瓣膜手术术后平均住院天数为7.5天（图3-3）。

The post-operative length of stay is one of the most important quality measures for valve surgery. The post-operative length of stay at Fuwai hospital was only 7.5 days（Figure 3-3）.

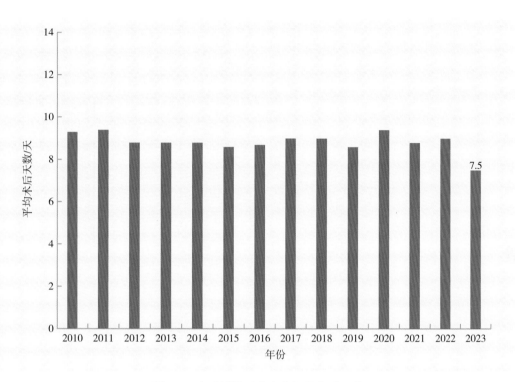

图3-3　心脏瓣膜手术患者平均术后天数

Figure 3-3　Postoperative length of stay of valvular heart surgery

► 典型病例

33岁男性患者，活动后胸闷症状3年，术前心脏超声提示主动脉瓣二瓣化畸形，主动脉瓣大量返流，左心室舒张末内径69mm，主动脉瓣环直径32mm，主动脉窦部直径39mm，升主动脉直径40mm。患者行胸骨上段小切口主动脉瓣修复手术，采用瓣环环缩＋瓣叶成形的综合修复策略，术后1年复查主动脉瓣功能正常。

二瓣化主动脉瓣关闭不全患者多为年轻患者，主动脉瓣修复手术可以保留自身主动脉瓣膜，避免了人工瓣膜置换相关并发症，术后患者生活质量与正常人一样。自2017年至今，二瓣化主动脉瓣修复手术124例，5年免于主动脉瓣二次手术率为95.64%，达到国际先进水平（图3-4）。

A 33-year-old male patient presented with chest tightness following physical exertion for three years. Preoperative echocardiography revealed bicuspid aortic valve, severe aortic valve regurgitation, left ventricular end-diastolic dimension is 69mm, aortic valve annulus diameter is 32mm, aortic sinus diameter is 39mm, and an ascending aorta diameter of 40mm. A minimally invasive aortic valve repair surgery via an upper sternal incision was performed, employing a comprehensive repair approach involving annuloplasty and valve repair. One-year post-surgery, the patient exhibited normal aortic valve function.

Individuals afflicted with BAV regurgitation are frequently young, and opting for aortic valve repair surgery can conserve the patient's native valve, eluding complications inherent in artificial valve replacement, thus enabling a quality of life akin to that of healthy individuals. Since 2017, Fuwai has performed 124 bicuspid aortic valve repair surgeries, a 5-year freedom from reoperation rate of 95.64%, attaining an internationally advanced standard.

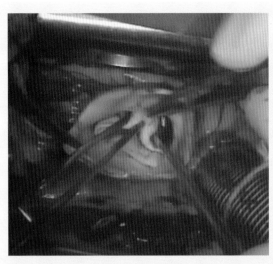

左右融合型二瓣化，交界角度 160°，瓣缘增厚
Bicuspid Type I LR，commissural angle 160°，thickened
Free margin

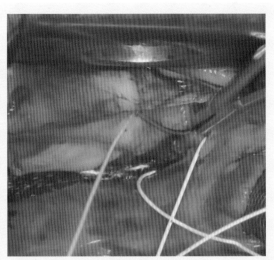

CV-0 缝线在基底环水平环缩瓣环
Annuloplasty at basal ring with CV-0

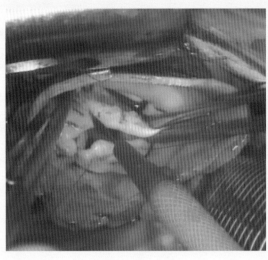

削薄增厚的游离缘
Shaving thickened Free margin

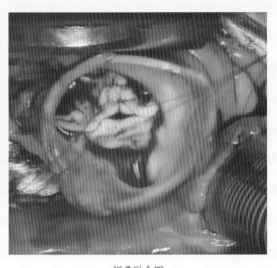

折叠融合瓣
Fusion cusp plication

图3-4　二瓣化主动脉瓣修复手术
Figure3-4　Bicuspid aortic valve repair

► 强化关键指标

2023年，二尖瓣成形术比例保持在瓣膜术种首位，主动脉瓣成形术比例稳定增加，这是阜外医院瓣膜综合修复技术的体现（图3-5）。

In 2023, mitral valve repair ranks the major proportion of all valvar surgeries. The aortic valve repair technique improved a lot as well, demonstrating the outstanding valve repairment technique at Fuwai hospital（Figure 3-5）.

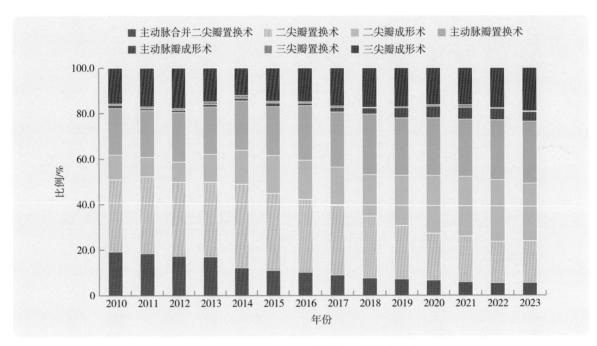

图3-5　2010—2023年心脏瓣膜手术种类构成

Figure 3-5　Types of valvular heart surgery, 2010—2023

　　瓣膜成形术手段越来越多，修复成功率稳步提高。阜外医院外科团队开展全面、规范、优质的瓣膜成形术，疗效显著。2023年，我院共完成单纯二尖瓣关闭不全患者的二尖瓣成形术907例，占比83.4%（图3-6）。

As our deep understanding of the structure and function of cardiac valves，the volume of valvuloplasty increases，with the improvement of repair rates. Fuwai Hospital can perform comprehensive，standardized and superior valve repairment procedures. In the year of 2023，907（83.4%）patients underwent surgical repairment procedures（Figure 3-6）.

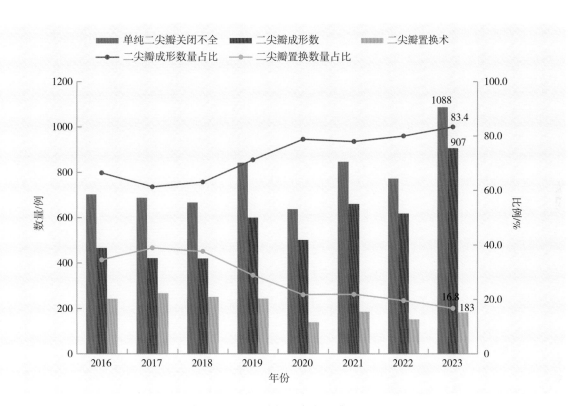

图3-6　2016—2023年单纯二尖瓣关闭不全中瓣膜成形术数量和置换术比例

Figure 3-6　Volume and proportion of surgical repairment procedures for isolated mitral valve insufficiency, 2010—2023

▶ 学术聚焦（表3-1）

表3-1 中国免缝合瓣膜临床研究（PERFECT）SuAVR和TAVR院内结果对比

变量	SuAVR（n=30）	TAVR（n=241）	P值
死亡（n/%）	0	9（3.7%）	0.03
开胸止血（n/%）	0	8（3.3%）	0.04
血滤（n/%）	0	1（0.4%）	0.75
卒中（n/%）	0	4（1.7%）	0.34
外周血管并发症（n/%）	0	7（2.9%）	0.04
永久起搏器植入（n/%）	1（4.3%）	37（15.4%）	0.02
瓣周漏（少量及以上）（n/%）	1（3.3%）	116（48.1%）	0.001
出院主动脉瓣峰值压差（mmHg）	17.0±6.5	31.2±14.2	0.04

注：SuAVR组在院内死亡、永久起搏器植入、瓣周漏等并发症以及血流动力学表现均优于TAVR组。

Complications such as in-hospital death，permanent pacemaker implantation，and perivalvular leakage were lower in the SuAVR group. The hemodynamic performance was better than that of the TAVR group.

● 设计开展对比复合消融与外科消融效果的随机对照研究
　RCT for comparison of hybrid ablation and surgical ablation
● 单中心随机对照研究，复合消融49例，外科消融48例，左房内径平均50.1mm（图3-7）。
　Hybrid ablation（n=49）vs Surgical ablation（n=48）（Figure 3-7）.

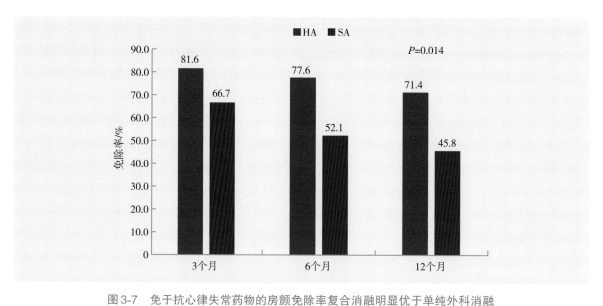

图3-7　免于抗心律失常药物的房颤免除率复合消融明显优于单纯外科消融

Figure 3-7　Antiarrhythmic drug-free and atrial fibrillation-free survival of hybrid ablation was significantly higher than surgical ablation

● 风湿性二尖瓣疾病合并房颤外科双房消融与左房消融疗效对比研究（ABLATION研究）（图3-8）。

Bi-atrial versus left atrial ablation for patients with rheumatic mitral valve disease and non-paroxysmal atrial fibrillation（ABLATION）

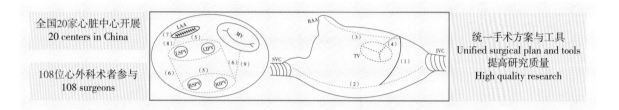

全国20家心脏中心开展
20 centers in China

108位心外科术者参与
108 surgeons

统一手术方案与工具
Unified surgical plan and tools
提高研究质量
High quality research

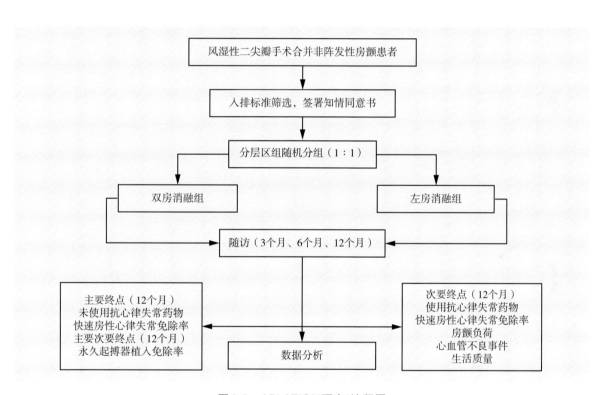

图3-8　ABLATION研究I流程图

Figure 3-8　The workflow of ABLATION Trial

研究目标

Objective

采用全国多中心随机对照研究，优化风湿性二尖瓣疾病合并房颤的外科消融方案。

A nationwide multicenter randomized controlled study to optimize the surgical ablation plan for rheumatic mitral valve disease with atrial fibrillation.

研究亮点

Highlights

1）采用中心分层随机化与中央随机系统，确保受试者分组均衡及隐匿，有效避免选择偏倚。

Central stratified randomization and central randomization system.

2）结合主要与次要终点的序贯检验策略，优化统计效能，提升研究严谨性。

Sequential testing strategy for primary and secondary endpoints to optimize statistical performance.

3）利用消融手术录像监测和多次Holter检测，保证操作标准化及终点采集准性，提高研究可靠性。

Utilizing video monitoring and multiple Holter tests to ensure standardized operation and accurate endpoint collection.

临床价值

Significance

1）针对临床诊疗突出问题，提供高等级循证证据，填补指南空白。

Providing high-level evidence-based evidence to fill the gap in guidelines.

2）多场学术会议培训，全国范围内推广标准房颤外科消融线路。

National promotion of standard atrial fibrillation surgical ablation.

四、主动脉及外周血管疾病外科治疗
Aortic and peripheral vascular diseases

▶ **概述**

2023年，阜外医院共完成主动脉外科手术治疗2248例，主动脉腔内支架修复手术685例（图4-1），均为历年来工作量最大的一年。本数据不包括小儿外科中心专家完成的小儿主动脉手术。

In 2023, there were 2248 open aortic surgery, and 685 endovascular aortic（Figure 4-1）. Both numbers are the largest annual volumes in history at Fuwai hospital. Our data do not include the aortic operations for infant and children performed at the Pediatric Cardiac Surgical Center.

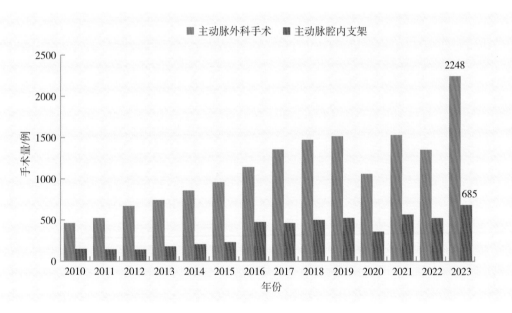

图4-1　2010—2023年主动脉外科手术量

Figure 4-1　Volume of aortic surgery, 2010—2023

图4-2显示了阜外医院血管外科历年以及2023年主动脉手术部位的构成情况。2023年患者构成比为，主动脉根部和升主动脉病变占31.6%，主动脉弓病变占35.4%，降主动脉病变占18.6%，胸腹主动脉病变占1.7%，腹主动脉病变占12.8%。

Figure 4-2 These figures show the composition of open，endovascular，and hybrid aortic procedures at Fuwai Hospital over the past several years. In 2023，31.6% of procedures were on the aortic root and ascending aorta，35.4% aortic arch，18.6% descending aorta，1.7% thoracoabdominal aorta，and 12.8% abdominal aorta.

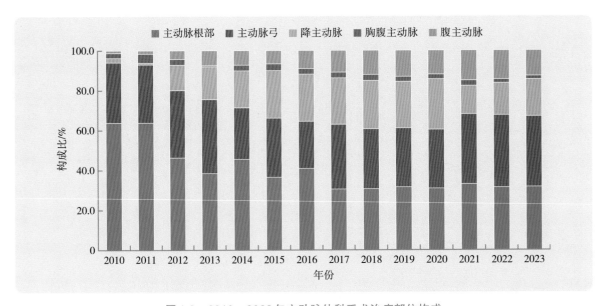

图4-2　2010—2023年主动脉外科手术治疗部位构成

Figure 4-2　Treatment region underwent aortic surgery, 2010—2023

近年来随着主动脉手术技术的发展和围手术期管理水平的提高，主动脉手术患者平均术后天数继续保持在较低水平。2023年主动脉手术患者平均术后天数7.3天（图4-3）。

In recent years，with the development of aortic surgery technology and the improvement of perioperative management，the average postoperative length of stay of aortic surgery patients remained at a low level. In 2023，the average postoperative length of stay of aortic surgery patients was 7.3 days（Figure 4-3）.

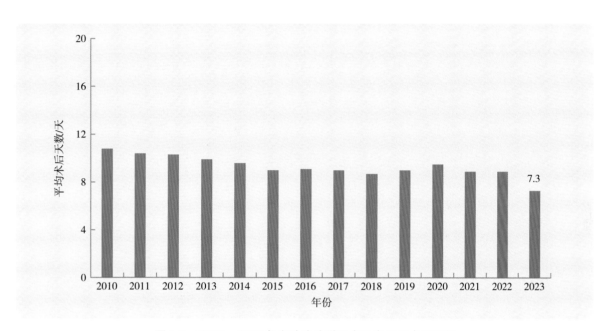

图4-3　2010—2023年主动脉外科手术患者平均术后天数

Figure 4-3　Post-operative length of stay, 2010—2023

2015年底，阜外医院血管外科中心重新组建外周血管疾病治疗团队，由血管外科中心一病区（血管外科医师和内科介入医师）、二病区（血管外科医师）组成，主要以外周动脉疾病介入和外科治疗作为主攻方向，兼顾静脉疾病。2023年，外周血管疾病治疗团队共实施手术2141例，30日死亡率为0，其中一病区、二病区的血管外科医师实施各类外周血管开放及介入手术1207例，内科介入医师实施外周血管介入手术934例。内科介入医师实施的外周动脉疾病和各类静脉疾病的介入手术量（934例）在阜外医院内科年报中体现，不计入阜外医院外科年报的心血管外科手术总量（图4-4）。

A dedicated peripheral vascular ward was established at Fuwai Hospital in November 2015. Ward staff include Team A vascular surgeons and Team B interventional cardiologists. In 2023, a total of 2141 peripheral vascular operations were performed, of which 1207 cases were performed by vascular surgeons in ward 1 and Ward 2, and 934 cases were performed by interventional cardiologists. The 30-day mortality is 0. The procedures performed by Team B（934 cases）were not included in the annual surgical volume of Fuwai Hospital（Figure 4-4）.

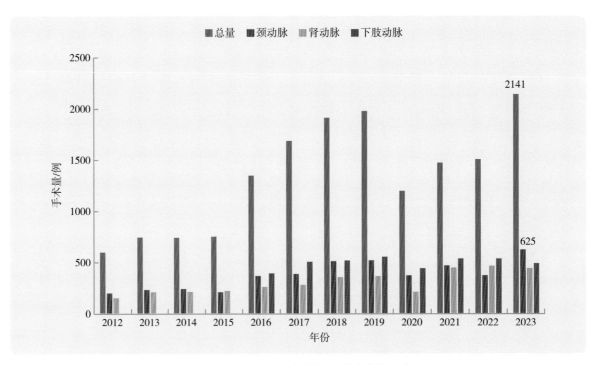

图4-4　2012—2023年周围血管疾病的治疗

Figure 4-4　Volume of peripheral vascular surgery, 2012—2023

2023年，在阜外医院血管外科中心完成的弓上动脉手术中，颈动脉手术占比最高，共完成625例，其中开放手术212例，介入手术413例。与前几年相比，颈动脉手术量明显增加（图4-5）。

In 2023, carotid artery surgeries accounted for the highest proportion of superior arch artery surgeries completed in the Vascular Surgery Center of Fuwai Hospital, with a total of 625 cases completed, including 212 CEA and 413 CAS. The volume of carotid artery surgeries significantly increased compared with previous years（Figure 4-5）.

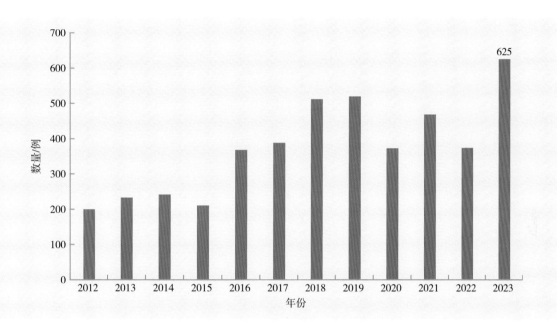

图4-5　2012—2023年颈动脉手术总量统计

Figure 4-5　Volume of carotid artery surgery, 2012—2023

► 典型病例

国产一体式单分支主动脉支架成功救治主动脉夹层破裂患者（图4-6）。

Single-branch aortic stentgraft for rupured aortic dissection（Figure 4-6）.

● 患者，男，59岁。

● 突发剧烈后背痛1天。

● 患者病情危急，入院后出现低氧血症（PaO$_2$ 66.2 mmHg）和中度贫血（HGB 66 g/L）。CTA提示Stanford B型主动脉夹层并破裂、纵膈及左侧胸腔大量积液、左侧肺不张，主动脉夹层破口累及弓部Z2和Z3区，且邻近左锁骨下动脉开口。

● 为抢救患者生命，遂急诊行一体式单分支主动脉支架植入术，在隔绝主动脉破口的同时保证左锁骨下动脉血供。

● 手术主体时间仅10分钟，手术时间均远远低于传统外科治疗，术后患者恢复良好。

● A 59-year-old male patient suffered from abrupt server backpain for 1 day, admitted with hypoxemia（PaO$_2$ 66.2 mmHg）and anemia（HGB 66 g/L）.

● CTA indicated Stanford type B aortic dissection with aortic rupture, mediastinum and left pleural effusion, and left pulmonary atelectasis. The aortic pathology involved Zone 2 and Zone 3, and was adjacent to the orifice of the left subclavian artery.

● In order to save the patient's life, the single-branch aortic stent-graft implantation was performed in emergency to isolate the aortic rupture and ensure the blood supply of the left subclavian artery.

● The X-ray exposure time（from first DSA to last DSA）was only 10 minutes, which was much lower than the traditional surgical treatment. The patient recovered well after operation.

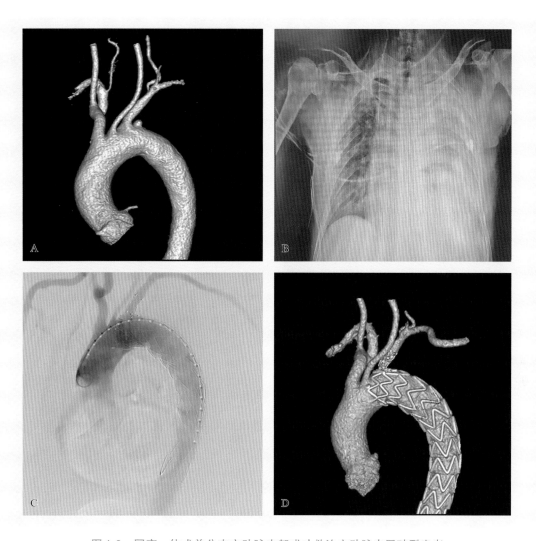

图4-6　国产一体式单分支主动脉支架成功救治主动脉夹层破裂患者

Figure 4-6　Single-branch Aortic Stent-graft for Ruptured Aortic Dissection

注：A.术前主动脉CT；B.胸部平片；C.术中造影图像；D.术后主动脉CT。

A. preoperative aortic CTA；B. Chest X-ray；C. intraoperative angiography images；D. postoperative aortic CTA .

▶ 强化关键指标

以急性主动脉综合征、主动脉破裂为代表的主动脉急症往往需要紧急手术，技术难度大，手术风险高。阜外医院集全院优势力量，从制度层面入手，建立了"胸痛中心"和"主动脉急诊绿色通道"，在主动脉急诊患者的救治效率和救治成功率方面，均已成为中国医院救治主动脉疾病的典范。2023年，阜外医院血管外科中心为1905例主动脉疾病患者实施了择期手术，为343例患者实施了急诊手术，术后30日死亡率分别低至0.2%和2.6%（院前死亡和急诊准备期间的术前死亡未统计在内）（图4-7）。

Aortic emergencies, including acute aortic syndrome and aortic rupture, are usually life-threatening, sudden onset catastrophes of the aorta that present immense surgical technique challenges and have high associated risks. The Aortic Emergency Green Channel policy of Fuwai Hospital has been in place for years and has helped ensure that the majority of emergent aortic patients are treated efficiently. The hospital continues to have one of the highest technical success rates for emergent aortic operations in the world. In 2023, surgeons at the Vascular Surgery Center performed 1, 905 scheduled surgeries and 343 emergent aortic surgeries, with 30-day mortality of 0.2% and 2.6%, respectively（deaths before hospital admission and during the preoperative preparation period in the emergency room were excluded from calculations）（Figure 4-7）.

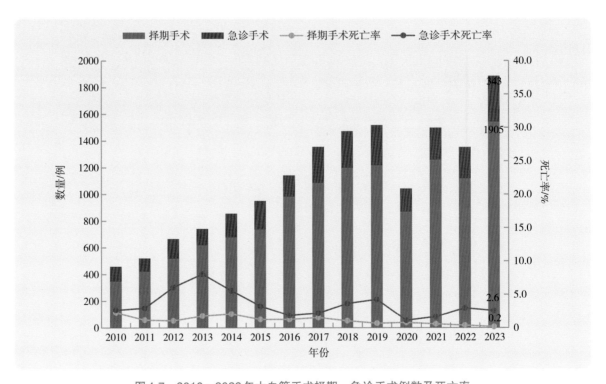

图4-7 2010—2023年大血管手术择期、急诊手术例数及死亡率

Figure 4-7 Volume and mortality of elective and emergency aortic surgery, 2010—2023

▶ 学术聚焦

主动脉弓部一体式三分支覆膜支架系统技术的临床应用（图4-8）。

Concave Supra-arch branched stent-graft system（Figure 4-8）.

该系统简化了主动脉弓部手术重建步骤和方式，有效缩短了手术时间，为广大医患提供了一种更简便的全腔内弓部病变微创修复方案，实现了主动脉弓部病变腔内治疗的突破。

The system simplifies the steps of surgical reconstruction of the aortic arch，effectively shortens the surgical time，achieving a breakthrough in endovascular treatment of aortic arch lesions.

2023年已完成FIM研究10例患者入组，大部分手术时间在1小时内。最长随访时间11个月，术后随访显示主动脉弓部及分支动脉与支架贴合良好，无不良事件发生。

In 2023，10 patients have been enrolled.Most of the surgerie took less than 1 hour. The hiaximum follow-up time was 11 months. The postoperative follow-up showed that the aortic arch and branch arteries were well fitted withthe stent，and no adverse events occurred.

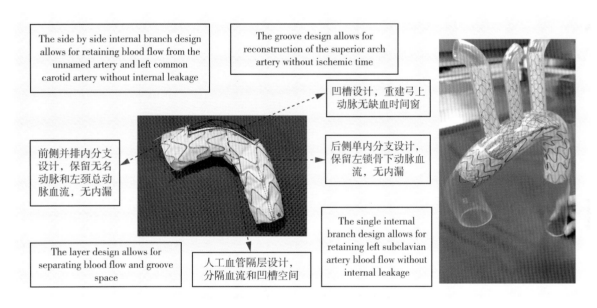

图4-8　主动脉弓部一体式三分支覆膜支架系统技术

Figure 4-8　Concave supra-arch branched stent-graft system

五、先天性心脏病外科治疗
Congenital Heart Diseases

▶ 概述

2023年，共完成先天性心脏病手术4660例，死亡率仅为0.2%（图5-1）。阜外医院小儿心脏外科中心2023年全年手术量已完全恢复至往年最高水平，同时在院死亡率保持进一步下降趋势，仅为0.2%。

In 2023, the volume of congenital heart surgeries was 4, 660, with an extremely low mortality of 0.2% (Figure 5-1). The Pediatric Cardiac Surgery Centre at Fuwai Hospital has fully recovered its annual surgical volume to its highest level of previous years by 2023. In addition, the in-hospital mortality rate has continued to decline to just 0.2%.

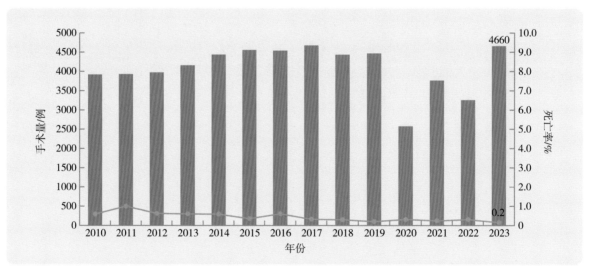

图5-1 2010—2023年先天性心脏病手术量及手术死亡率

Figure 5-1 Volume and mortality of congenital heart surgery, 2010—2023

2023年由国家心血管病中心、中国医学科学院阜外医院发起并成立国家心血管病中心先天性心脏病一体化专科联盟，以提升先天性心脏病危重症救治能力。在该联盟的支持下，环京津冀多个省市的复杂危重先天性心脏病患儿得到了更及时、有效的救治。2023年阜外医院危重复杂先天性心脏病手术量达到3610例，创历史新高（图5-2）。新生儿心脏手术死亡率维持低水平（图5-3）。

In 2023, The Centre of National Cardiovascular Disease（NCVDC）and Fuwai Hospital, the Chinese Academy of Medical Sciences（CAMS）initiated and established the National Cardiovascular Disease Centre Specialist Alliance for the Integration of Congenital Heart Disease to enhance the capacity of critical care for congenital heart disease. With the support of this alliance, children with complex and critical congenital heart disease in many provinces and cities around Beijing, Tianjin and Hebei have received more timely and effective treatment. The number of critical and complex congenital heart disease surgeries at Fuwai Hospital reached a record high of 3，610 cases in 2023（Figure 5-2）. Neohatal cardiac sugery mortality remains low（Figure 5-3）.

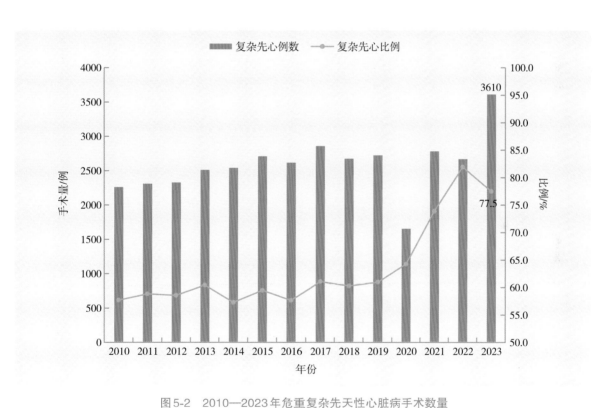

图5-2　2010—2023年危重复杂先天性心脏病手术数量

Figure 5-2　Volume of critical and complex corgenital heare Surgery, 2010—2023

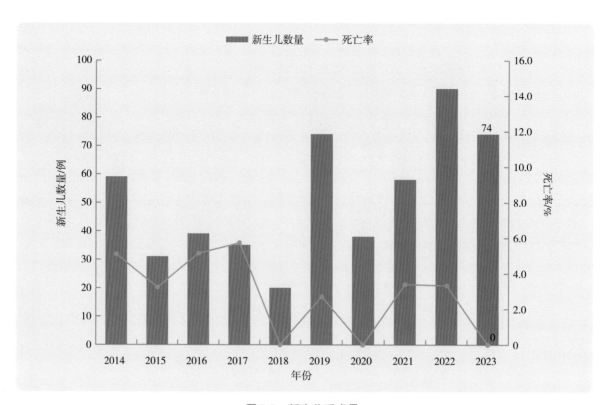

图5-3 新生儿手术量

Figure 5-3 Volume of neonatal cardiac surgery

3岁以下先天性心脏病患儿的比例连续第3年下降。而大于14岁的先天性心脏病患儿比例连续稳定在20%以上，这体现了在术后的先天性心脏病患者数量逐年累积下，众多大龄儿童患者需接受再次手术（图5-4）。随着术后时间的进一步增加，大龄儿童、成人的先天性心脏病再次手术可能成为未来先天性心脏病外科治疗的新趋势。

For the third year in a row, the proportion of children with congenital heart disease under the age of 3 has decreased. However, the proportion of children with congenital heart disease over the age of 14 has remained stable at over 20% for consecutive years, reflecting the need for reoperation for many older children as the number of post-operative congenital heart disease patients increases each year (Figure 5-4). With further increases in postoperative time, reoperation for congenital heart disease in older children and adults may become a new trend in the future surgical treatment of congenital heart disease.

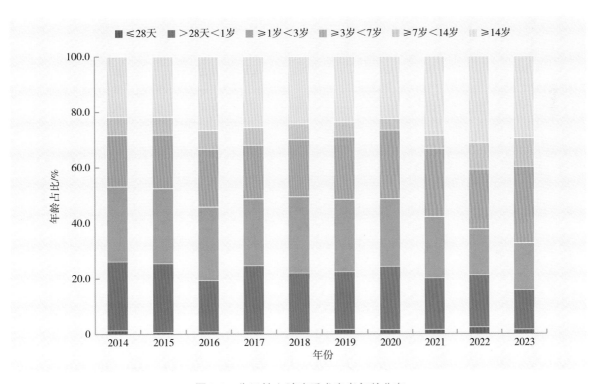

图5-4　先天性心脏病手术患者年龄分布

Figure 5-4　Age distribution of congenital heart surgery

在外科、重症医学科、麻醉科、体外循环科、超声科等多学科共同努力下，小儿中心的医疗质量进一步提升，体现在平均住院天数连续第3年下降，仅为7.2天（图5-5）。

The multidisciplinary efforts of the departments of surgery, intensive care, anesthesia, extracorporeal circulation and ultrasound have resulted in a further improvement in the quality of care at the Children's Centre, as evidenced by a reduction in the average length of stay for the third consecutive year to 7.2 days and a significant reduction in the cost of hospitalization (Figure 5-5).

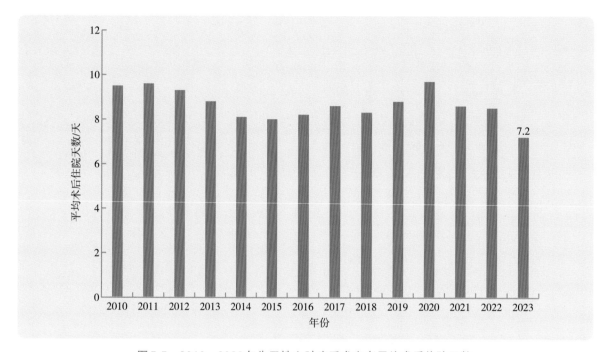

图5-5　2010—2023年先天性心脏病手术患者平均术后住院天数
Figure 5-5　Postoperative length of stay of congenital heart surgery, 2010—2023

▶ **典型病例**

Potts分流术又称为降主动脉-肺动脉连结术（图5-6），是降主动脉直接或通过带瓣/不带瓣的人工管道吻合到左肺动脉，人为构建体肺循环通道，降低右心室后负荷，造成"艾森曼格综合症"的血流动力学状态，改善患者肺动脉高压症状，延长患者寿命。国际上，Potts分流术多用于终末期肺动脉高压过度肺移植的姑息性治疗手段，研究表明Potts分流术的6年生存率与肺移植没有明显差异。本中心目前已成功开展Potts分流术用于终末期肺动脉高压肺移植的桥接治疗，取得良好临床效果。

Potts shunt, also known as descending aorta-pulmonary artery connection (Figure 5-6), involves anastomosing the descending aorta directly or through valved/unvalved artificial conduits to the left pulmonary artery to create an artificial systemic-to-pulmonary circulation pathway. This procedure reduces the afterload on the right ventricle, creating a hemodynamic state similar to Eisenmenger syndrome, improving symptoms of pulmonary arterial hypertension, and extending patient lifespan. Internationally, Potts shunt is mostly used as a palliative treatment for end-stage pulmonary arterial hypertension prior to lung transplantation. Studies have shown that the 6-year survival rate of Potts shunt is not significantly different from lung transplantation. Our center has successfully performed Potts shunt as a bridging treatment for end-stage pulmonary arterial hypertension before lung transplantation, achieving good clinical outcomes.

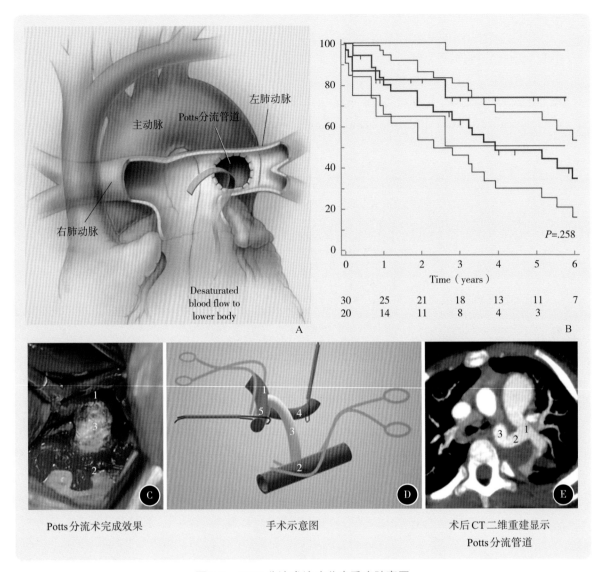

图5-6　Potts分流术治疗儿童重度肺高压

Figure 5-6　Potts shunt for the treatment of pulmonary hypertension in children

注：1：左肺动脉，2：降主动脉，3：Potts分流管道，4：左上肺动脉，5：左下肺动脉

► **学术聚焦**

中国先天性心脏病系列论文（图5-7）。

The Lancet Child & Adolescent Health–Series（Figure 5-7）.

● 中国先天性心脏病治疗现状及未来展望

● Current treatment outcomes and future perspectives

● 中国先天性心脏病外科手术经济负担

● Economic burden of congenital heart surgery in China

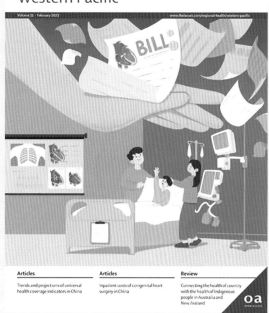

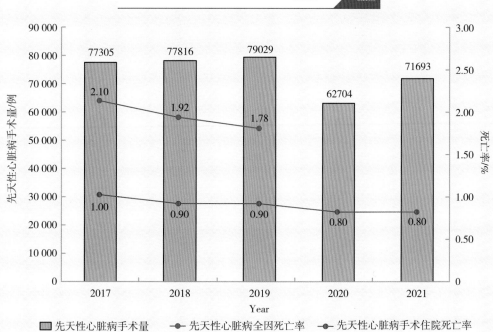

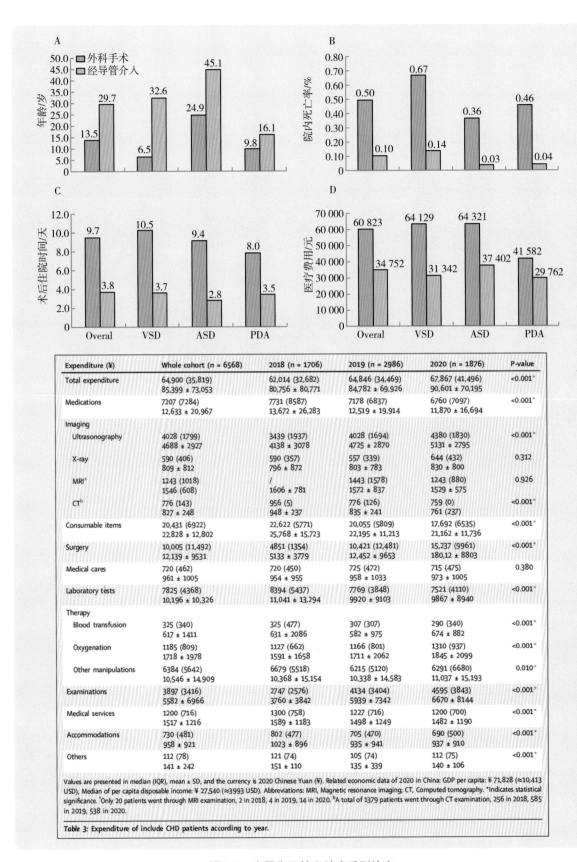

Expenditure (¥)	Whole cohort (n = 6568)	2018 (n = 1706)	2019 (n = 2986)	2020 (n = 1876)	P-value
Total expenditure	64,900 (35,819) 85,399 ± 73,053	62,014 (32,682) 80,756 ± 80,771	64,846 (34,469) 84,782 ± 69,926	67,867 (41,496) 90,601 ± 70,195	<0.001*
Medications	7207 (7284) 12,633 ± 20,967	7731 (8587) 13,672 ± 26,283	7178 (6837) 12,519 ± 19,914	6760 (7097) 11,870 ± 16,694	<0.001*
Imaging					
Ultrasonography	4028 (1799) 4688 ± 2927	3439 (1937) 4138 ± 3078	4028 (1694) 4725 ± 2870	4380 (1830) 5131 ± 2795	<0.001*
X-ray	590 (406) 809 ± 812	590 (357) 796 ± 872	557 (339) 803 ± 783	644 (432) 830 ± 800	0.312
MRI[a]	1243 (1018) 1546 (608)	/ 1606 ± 781	1443 (1578) 1572 ± 837	1243 (880) 1529 ± 575	0.926
CT[b]	776 (143) 827 ± 248	956 (5) 948 ± 237	776 (126) 835 ± 241	759 (0) 761 (237)	<0.001*
Consumable items	20,431 (6922) 22,828 ± 12,802	22,622 (5771) 25,768 ± 15,723	20,055 (5809) 22,195 ± 11,213	17,692 (6535) 21,162 ± 11,736	<0.001*
Surgery	10,005 (11,492) 12,139 ± 9531	4851 (1354) 5133 ± 3779	10,421 (12,481) 12,452 ± 9653	15,237 (9961) 180,12 ± 8803	<0.001*
Medical cares	720 (462) 961 ± 1005	720 (450) 954 ± 955	725 (472) 958 ± 1033	715 (475) 973 ± 1005	0.380
Laboratory tests	7825 (4368) 10,196 ± 10,326	8394 (5437) 11,041 ± 13,294	7769 (3848) 9920 ± 9103	7521 (4110) 9867 ± 8940	<0.001*
Therapy					
Blood transfusion	325 (340) 617 ± 1411	325 (477) 631 ± 2086	307 (307) 582 ± 975	290 (340) 674 ± 882	<0.001*
Oxygenation	1185 (809) 1718 ± 1978	1127 (662) 1591 ± 1658	1166 (801) 1711 ± 2062	1310 (937) 1845 ± 2099	<0.001*
Other manipulations	6384 (5642) 10,546 ± 14,909	6679 (5518) 10,368 ± 15,154	6215 (5120) 10,338 ± 14,583	6291 (6680) 11,037 ± 15,193	0.010*
Examinations	3897 (3416) 5582 ± 6966	2747 (2576) 3760 ± 3842	4134 (3404) 5939 ± 7342	4595 (3843) 6670 ± 8144	<0.001*
Medical services	1200 (716) 1517 ± 1216	1300 (758) 1589 ± 1183	1227 (716) 1498 ± 1249	1200 (700) 1482 ± 1190	<0.001*
Accommodations	730 (481) 958 ± 921	802 (477) 1023 ± 896	705 (470) 935 ± 941	690 (500) 937 ± 910	<0.001*
Others	112 (78) 141 ± 242	121 (74) 151 ± 110	105 (74) 135 ± 339	112 (75) 140 ± 106	<0.001*

Values are presented in median (IQR), mean ± SD, and the currency is 2020 Chinese Yuan (¥). Related economic data of 2020 in China: GDP per capita: ¥ 71,828 (≈10,413 USD), Median of per capita disposable income: ¥ 27,540 (≈3993 USD). Abbreviations: MRI, Magnetic resonance imaging; CT, Computed tomography. *Indicates statistical significance. [a]Only 20 patients went through MRI examination, 2 in 2018, 4 in 2019, 14 in 2020. [b]A total of 1379 patients went through CT examination, 256 in 2018, 585 in 2019, 538 in 2020.

Table 3: Expenditure of include CHD patients according to year.

图 5-7 中国先天性心脏病系列论文

Figure 5-7 The Lancet Child & Adolescent Health-Series

国家支持成立先心病一体化专科联盟（图5-8）。

Prenatal diagnosis and postnatal treatment integrated model with national support（Figure 5-8）.

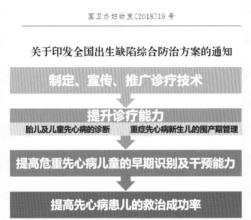

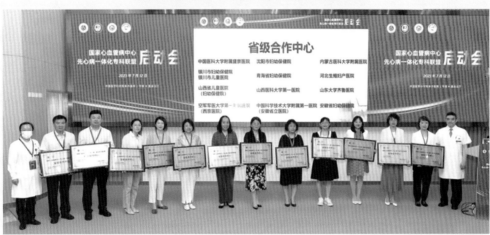

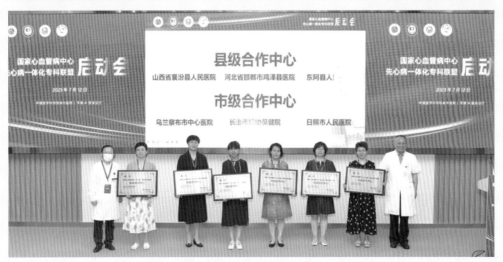

图5-8　国家支持成立先心病一体化专科联盟

Figure 5-8　Prenatal diagnosis and postnatal treatment integrated model with national support

改良L型切口法治疗完全性肺静脉异位引流（图5-9）。

Modified L-shaped incision in TAPVC repair（Figure 5-9）.

International Journal of Surgery 发表论文

International Journal of Surgery-Research article

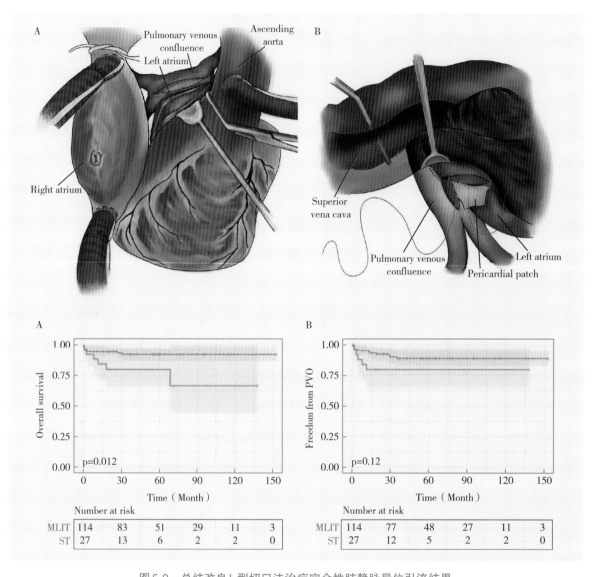

图5-9　总结改良L型切口法治疗完全性肺静脉异位引流结果

Figure 5-9　Reporting outcomes of modified L-shaped incision treating TAPVC

六、结构性心脏病外科治疗
Structural heart diseases

▶ **概述**

经导管主动脉瓣置换术（transcatheter aortic valve replacement，TAVR）是近十年逐渐兴起的微创主动脉瓣置换术，有经导管与经心尖两种释放方式。随着国际上TAVR的适应证逐渐放宽，TAVR已经成为主动脉瓣置换的主流术式之一。阜外医院2023年共完成498例TAVR，其中外科完成270例，另有48例经心尖TAVR由外科独立完成（图6-1）。

Transcatheter aortic valve replacement（TAVR）is a minimally invasive aortic valve replacement that has emerged in the last decade, with both transcatheter and transapical delivery. With the gradual relaxation of international indications for TAVR, it has become one of the mainstream procedures for aortic valve replacement. A total of 498 cases of TAVR were completed at Fuwai Hospital in 2023, of which 270 cases were completed by surgeons. Besides, there are another 48 cases of transapical TAVR were completed independently by surgeons（Figure 6-1）.

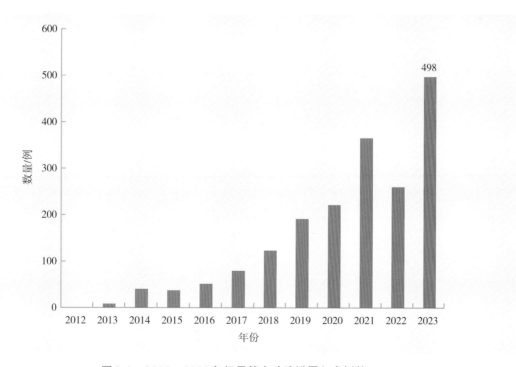

图6-1　2012—2023年经导管主动脉瓣置入术例数

Figure 6-1　Volume of transcatheter aortic valve replacement, 2012—2023

二尖瓣反流是最常见的心脏瓣膜疾病。近年来，二尖瓣病变经导管介入治疗得到了极大的发展，主要包括经导管二尖瓣修复术和经导管二尖瓣置换术（TMVR）。经导管二尖瓣修复术主要包括瓣叶修复、瓣环成型和腱索修复等。阜外医院2023年共完成介入二尖瓣手术76例，其中介入二尖瓣修复67例，介入二尖瓣置换9例（图6-2）。

Mitral regurgitation is the most common heart valve disease. In recent years, transcatheter intervention therapy for mitral valve disease has made great progress, mainly including transcatheter mitral valve repair and transcatheter mitral valve replacement（TMVR）. Transcatheter mitral valve repair mainly includes leaflet repair, annulus formation, and chordae tendineae repair. In 2023, Fuwai Hospital completed a total of 76 cases of interventional mitral valve surgery, including 67 cases of interventional mitral valve repair and 9 cases of interventional mitral valve replacement（Figure 6-2）.

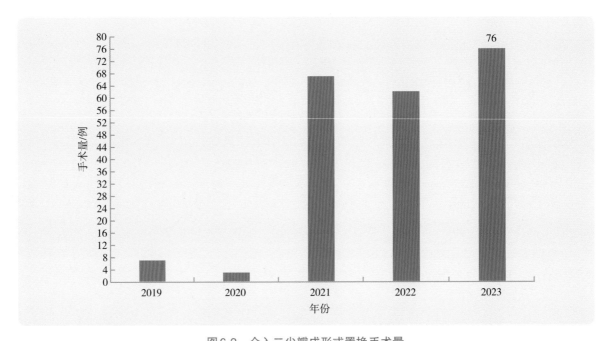

图6-2　介入二尖瓣成形或置换手术量

Figure 6-2　Volume of transcatheter mitral valve repair or replacement

先天性心脏病矫治术后肺动脉瓣大量反流患者往往需要进行经皮肺动脉瓣植入术，经皮肺动脉瓣植入术是解剖结构合适患者的首选手段。国内患者存在右心室流出道瘤样扩张的独特解剖特征，国际常用的球扩瓣往往不适合国内患者，尤其是右心室流出道过大的患者。目前，国内自主研发的自膨肺动脉瓣已完成临床试验并于2022年获得NMPA批准于中国上市。2023年阜外医院共完成经皮肺动脉瓣植入术36例（图6-3）。

Patients with severe pulmonary valve regurgitation after congenital heart disease correction surgery often require percutaneous pulmonary valve implantation, which is the preferred method for patients with appropriate anatomical structure. Patients in China have unique anatomical features of right ventricular outflow tract tumor like dilation, and internationally commonly used balloon valves are often not suitable for Chinese patients, especially those with large right ventricular outflow tract. At present, the domestically independently developed self expanding pulmonary artery valve has completed clinical trials and obtained NMPA approval for listing in China in 2022. In 2023, a total of 36 cases of percutaneous pulmonary valve implantation were completed in Fuwai Hospital (Figure 6-3).

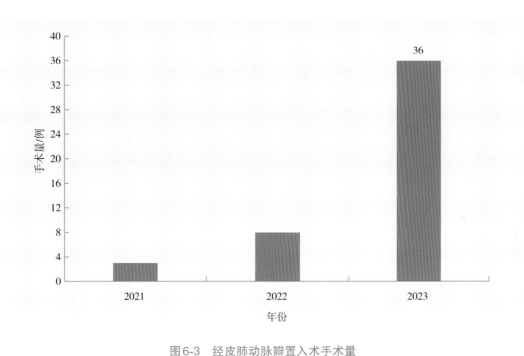

图6-3　经皮肺动脉瓣置入术手术量

Figure 6-3　Volume of percutaneous pulmonary valve implantation

▶ 典型病例

　　常规开展纯超声引导经导管二尖瓣缘对缘修复技术（MitraClip），阜外结构团队率先使用纯超声引导技术完成Mitraclip手术，并通过线上线下相结合的多场教学直播，将阜外技术向外推广（图6-4）。

　　Rim-to-rim transcatheter mitral valve repair is routinely performed by ultrasound guidance. Fuwai team of structural heart disease was the first to perform the Mitraclip procedure by only using ultrasound guidance and has promoted Fuwai's technology to the outside world through a series of live online and offline teaching sessions（Figure 6-4）.

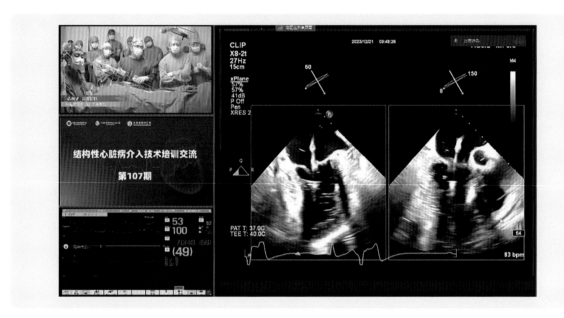

图6-4　共举办27期Mitraclip手术教学直播

Figure 6-4　A total of 27 live Mitraclip surgical training sessions were held

► **学术聚焦**

原创心血管器械标志成果举例——可吸收封堵器研发（图6-5）。

Resorbable Occluder-Examples of Original Cardiovascular Device Markers（Figure 6-5）.

- 可吸收封堵器的困境：无法完全吸收。
- 可吸收材料在放射线下不显影。
- 传统技术在放射线下才能植入封堵器。
- 需在可吸收封堵器上增加金属标记物。
- 可吸收材料吸收后金属标记脱落栓塞。
- The dilemma of the absorbable blocker is incomplete absorption.
- Absorbable materials are not visible under radiation.
- The radiation is necessary to implant an occlude by traditional technique.
- Additional metal markers are required for resorbable occluder.
- Metal markers are easily dislodged and can cause emboli.

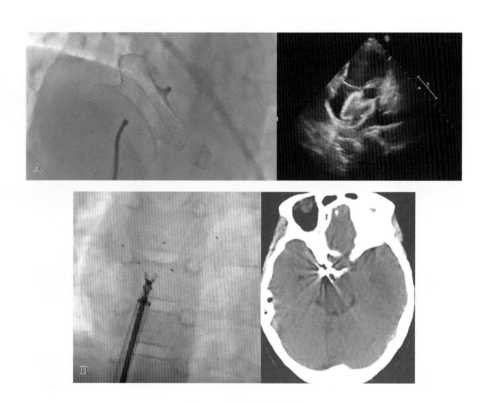

图6-5 可吸收封堵器

Figure 6-5 Resorbable Occluder

注：A.传统镍钛合金封堵器；B.添加金属标记的非完全可吸收封堵器。

A. Conventional Nitinol Occluder；B. Non-fully Absorbable Occluder with Metal Markers.

超声引导介入技术可以植入完全可吸收封堵器。持续引领全球完全可吸收封堵器研发（图6-6，图6-7）。开创了一个新的医疗器械序列。

Ultrasound-guided procedures allow implantation of fully resorbable occluder. To continue to be the world leader in the development of fully resorbable occluder(Figure 6-6, Figure 6-7). Created a new medical device sequence.

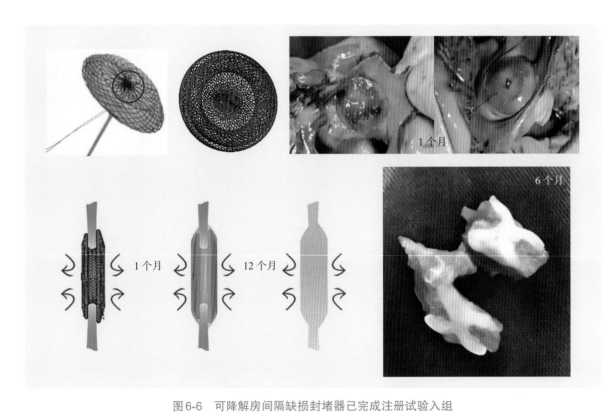

图6-6　可降解房间隔缺损封堵器已完成注册试验入组

Figure 6-6　The biodegradable atrial septal defect occluder has been enrolled into a pivotal trial

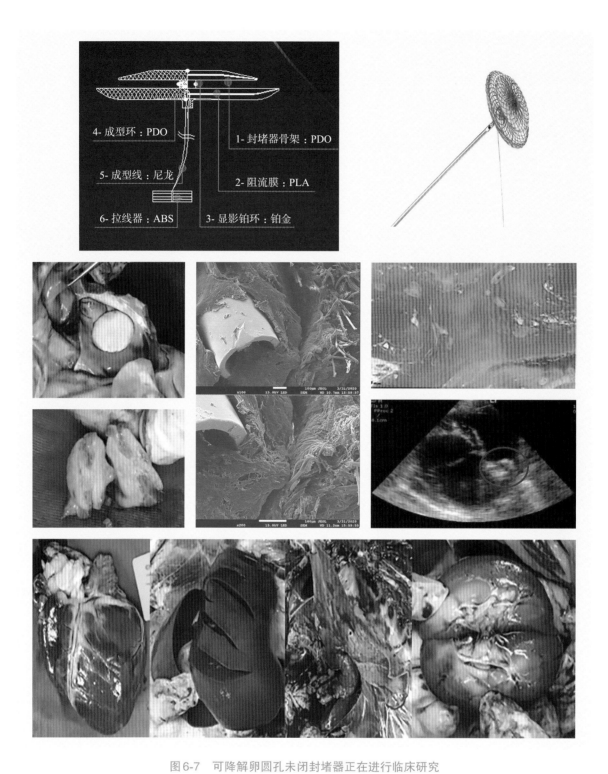

4- 成型环：PDO

1- 封堵器骨架：PDO

5- 成型线：尼龙

2- 阻流膜：PLA

6- 拉线器：ABS

3- 显影铂环：铂金

图6-7　可降解卵圆孔未闭封堵器正在进行临床研究

Figure 6-7　We are conducting a clinical trial of a biodegradable foramen oval occluder

超声引导移动手术车，实现"家庭作业式"的一站式治疗（图6-8）。

Ultrasound guided mobile surgical vehicle for "homework style" one-stop treatment（Figure 6-8）.

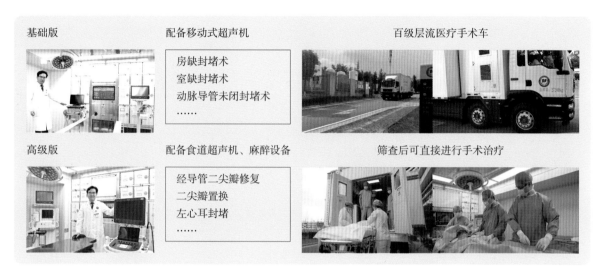

图6-8　方法学创新实现技术突破带动诊疗方式变革

Figure 6-8　Methodology innovation achieves technological breakthroughs and drives the transformation of diagnosis and treatment methods

召开第五届中国结构性心脏病大会及常态化培训（图6-9）。

The 5th China Structural Heart Disease Conference and regular training（Figure 6-9）.

● 召开第五届中国结构性心脏病大会：线上+线下的形式，参会人数近80000人。

● 线上手术直播：2023年已开展40场线上手术直播，邀请国内外100多位专家。

● 培训会议：召开2场线下培训会议，受培训人员超过3万人。

● 全国结构性心脏病介入技术培训基地：2023年共招收33名国内学员，2名外籍学员。

● Convening the 5th China Structural Heart Disease Conference: Online and offline，with nearly 80000 attendees.

● Online surgical live streaming: 40 online surgical live broadcasts，inviting more than 100 domestic and foreign experts.

● Training meetings: Two offline training meetings were held，with over 30000 trainees.

● The National Structural Heart Disease Intervention Technology Training Base: 33 domestic students and 2 foreign students.

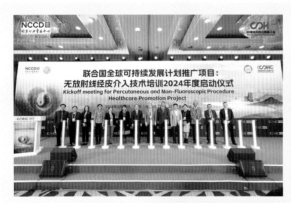
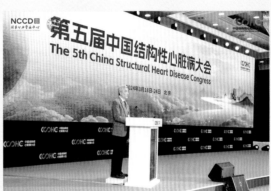
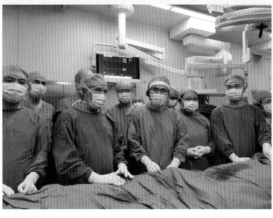

图6-9 第五届中国结构性心脏病大会及常态化培训

Figure 6-9 The 5th China Structural Heart Disease Conference and regular training

七、晚期心脏病外科治疗
Surgical treatment of late-stage heart disease

▶ 心脏移植

原位心脏移植术目前仍然是各类终末期心脏病的最有效治疗方案。阜外医院从供心的获取和保存，手术过程中外科、体外循环、麻醉的密切配合，以及术后的监护和康复等各个诊疗环节均形成了完整、高效、高质量的闭环。2023年，完成141例原位心脏移植手术，死亡率连续3年下降至1%以下（图7-1）。

In situ heart transplantation remains the most effective treatment option for all types of end-stage heart disease. Fuwai Hospital has established a complete, efficient and high-quality closed loop in all aspects of treatment, from the acquisition and preservation of the donor heart, to the close coordination of surgery, extracorporeal circulation and anesthesia during surgery, and postoperative monitoring and rehabilitation. In 2023, the total number of in situ heart transplants reached 141, with thc mortality ratc falling to less than 1% for the third consecutive year (Figure 7-1).

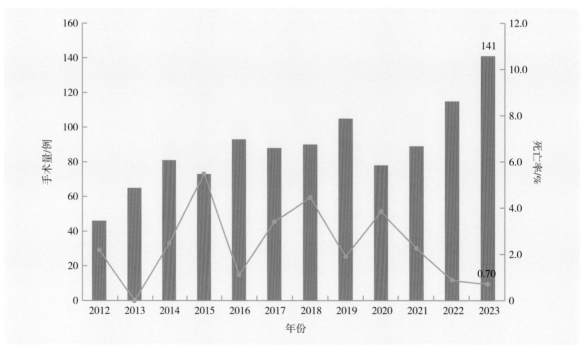

图7-1　2012—2023年心脏移植手术量

Figure 7-1　Volume of heart transplantation

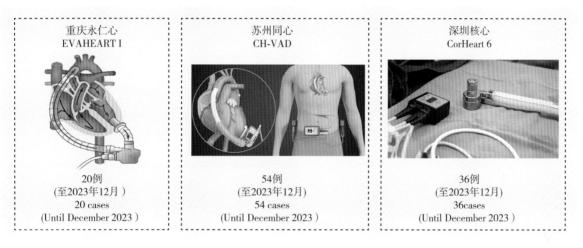

▶ 左心室辅助装置

阜外医院完成了全国最大规模的植入式左心室辅助装置（LVAD）的临床应用评价（图7-2）。

Fuwai Hospital has completed the clinical evaluation of the largest cohort of implantable left ventricular assist device（LVAD）in China（Figure 7-2）.

图7-2　植入式左心室辅助装置的临床应用

Figure 7-2　clinical application of left ventricular assist device

截至2023年12月，共完成110例LVAD植入。

Until December 2023，a total of 110 LVAD surgeries have been completed in Fuwai Hospital.

阜外医院LVAD治疗效果达到国际领先水平（表7-1）。

The outcome has reached the international leading level（Table 7-1）.

● 阜外医院单中心LVAD患者3年生存率优于国际应用最广泛的HM3辅助泵。

● 治疗效果接近国内心脏移植效果，达到国际领先水平。

● The 3-year survival rate of LVAD patients in Fuwai Hospital is better than that of Heatmate Ⅲ.

● The 3-year survival rate of LVAD patients in Fuwai Hospital is close to that of heart transplantation in China，reaching leading level around the world.

表7-1　植入式左心室辅助装置的临床应用评价

Table 7-1　Clinical evaluation of implantable left ventricular assist device

	HM3 （ n=177 ）	HTX （ n=344 ）	阜外LVAD （ n=100 ）	阜外HTX （ n=1096 ）
年龄（岁）	59（50～75）	50（38～59）	47（13～73）	55（12～67）
中位随访时间（天）	659（338～969）	710（391～1009）	646（44～2360）	1100（365～3275）
生存率				
1年	93%	92%	94.3%	94%
2年	87%	85%	90.6%	92%
3年	82%	85%	87.9%	91%

▶ Morrow 手术

针对梗阻性肥厚型心肌病，阜外医院 Morrow 手术稳定成熟。2023年全年全部 Morrow 手术无手术死亡和严重并发症，术后左心室流出道压差和室间隔厚度较术前显著（图 7-3）。

For hypertrophic obstructive cardiomyopathy，Morrow surgery at Fuwai Hospital is stable and mature. In 2023, there were no surgical deaths or serious complications in all Morrow surgeries，and the postoperative left ventricular outflow tract pressure difference and interventricular septal thickness were significantly higher than before（Figure 7-3）.

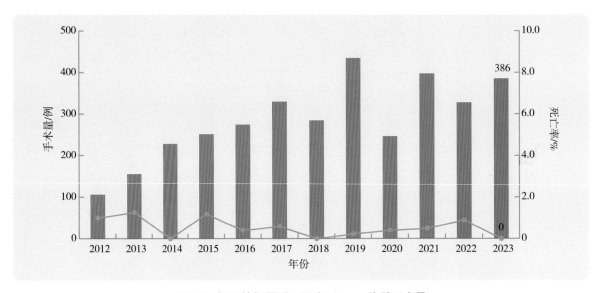

图7-3　梗阻性肥厚型心肌病 Morrow 外科手术量

Figure 7-3　Volume of Morrow procedure

▶ 肺栓塞

阜外医院开展肺动脉内膜剥脱术（PEA）手术以来，手术疗效达到国际领先水平。并在国内率先开展杂交技术（肺动脉内膜剥脱＋肺动脉球囊扩张术）治疗慢性血栓栓塞性肺动脉高压，为开展此类治疗方案的全球最大中心之一（图7-4）。

Since the implementation of pulmonary endarterectomy (PEA) surgery at Fuwai Hospital, the surgical efficacy has reached the international leading level. And it is the first in China to carry out hybrid technology (pulmonary artery intimal dissection+pulmonary artery balloon dilation) to treat chronic thromboembolic pulmonary hypertension, becoming one of the world's largest centers for such treatment plans (Figure 7-4).

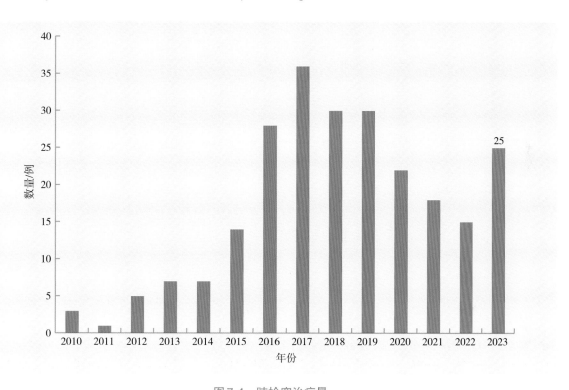

图7-4 肺栓塞治疗量

Figure 7-4 Volume of pulmonary endarterectomy

► **学术聚焦**

在国家自然基金委重大项目支持下异种移植项目稳步向前（图7-5～图7-8）。

Supported by major projects of the National Natural Science Foundation of China（Figure 7-5 ～ Figure 7-8）.

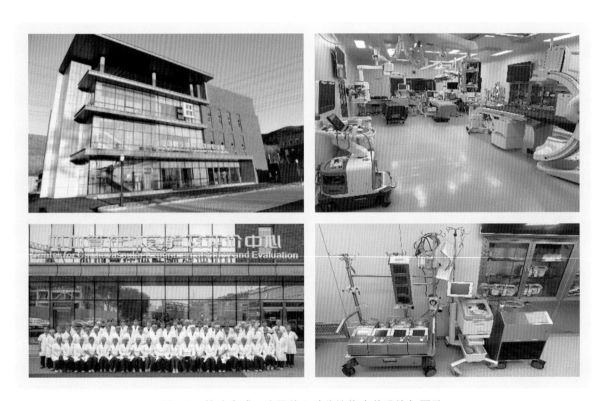

图7-5　构建全球一流异种心脏移植临床前设施与团队
Figure 7-5　Building world-class preclinical facilities and teams for xenograft heart transplantation

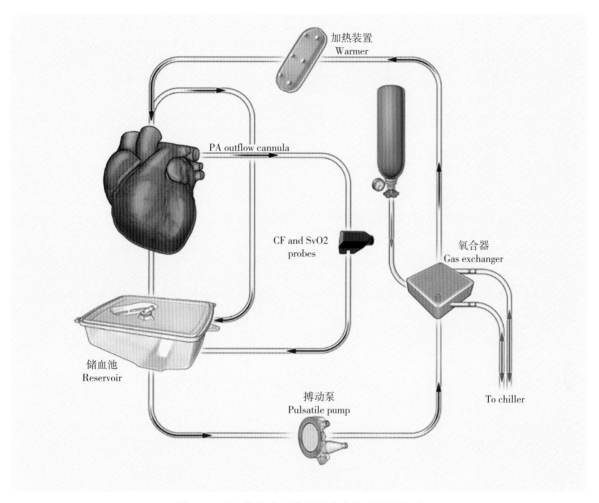

加热装置
Warmer

PA outflow cannula

CF and SvO2
probes

氧合器
Gas exchanger

储血池
Reservoir

To chiller

搏动泵
Pulsatile pump

图7-6　建立体外人血灌流亚临床快速评价体系

Figure 7-6　Establishing a subclinical rapid evaluation system for in vitro human blood perfusion

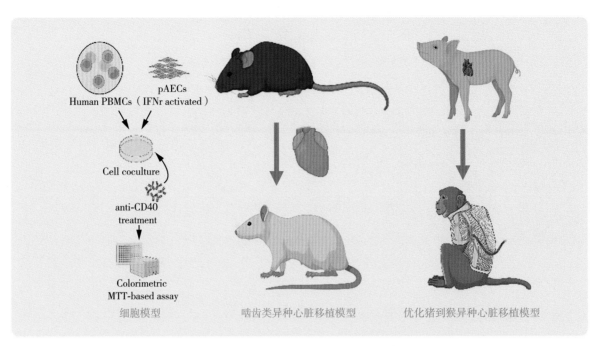

图7-7　建立从细胞到小动物再到大动物的免疫药物评价系统

Figure 7-7　Establishing an immune drug evaluation system from cells to small animals and then to large animals

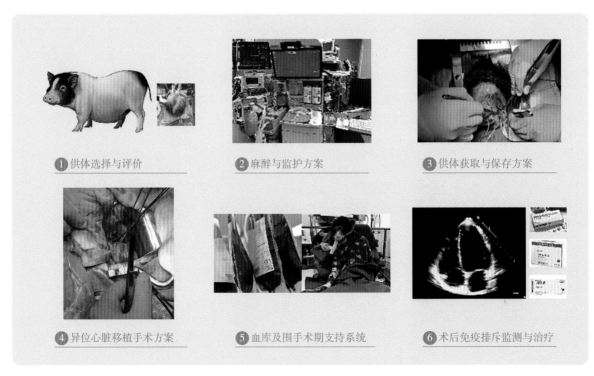

图7-8　构建长期稳定的猪到猴异种心脏移植模型

Figure 7-8　Constructing a long-term stable pig to monkey xenograft heart transplantation model

八、术后患者的全程康复和
生活方式医学的推广
Whole perioperative period cardiac rehabilitation and promotion of lifestyle medicine

▶ 外科围手术期的全程康复

心脏康复贯穿于心脏外科围手术期的全周期。从患者入院开始，既开始预康复，提高术前身体功能，减少术后并发症。患者手术后，从ICU开始早期康复。转回病房后，患者将延续康复训练，逐步提高活动水平，直至出院。术后3个月后，患者可至心脏康复门诊开展以运动、营养、睡眠、呼吸、心理为核心的二期康复，优化患者的体能和身体状态，完成疾病的二级预防，提高生活质量，并终身保持健康生活方式（图8-1）。

Cardiac rehabilitation runs through the whole perioperative period of cardiac surgery. Since the patient was admitted to the hospital, he has started pre-rehabilitation, improved preoperative physical function and reduced postoperative complications. After the operation, the patient began early rehabilitation from ICU. After being transferred back to the ward, the patient will continue rehabilitation training and gradually improve his activity level until he is discharged. Three months after operation, patients can go to the cardiac rehabilitation clinic to carry out the second-stage rehabilitation with exercise, nutrition, sleep, breathing and psychology as the core, optimize the physical fitness and physical state of patients, complete the secondary prevention of diseases, improve the quality of life and maintain a healthy lifestyle for life（Figure 8-1）.

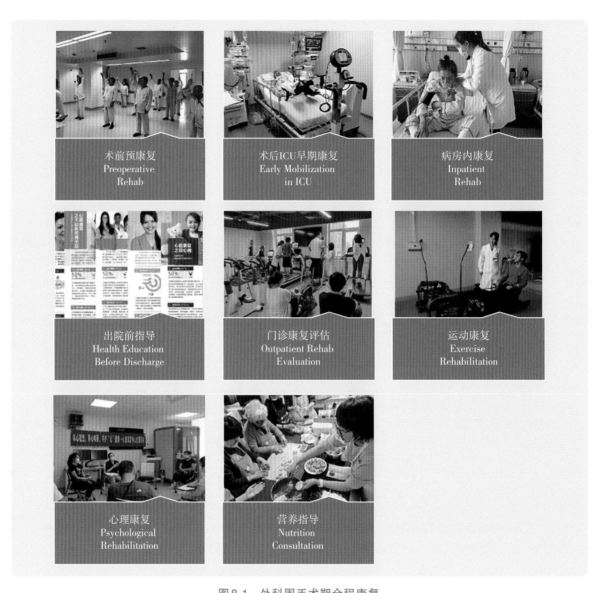

图8-1　外科围手术期全程康复

Figure 8-1　Perioperative rehabilitation of surgery

2023年，心脏康复中心完成了所有外科重症病房及外科普通病房的康复覆盖。

In 2023，Fuwai cardiac rehabilitation center covered the rehabilitation of all surgical intensive care units and surgical general wards.

将心外科围手术期康复拓展到成人外科病房、血管外科病房、结构病房、小儿外科病房、外科术后SICU等19个病区，干预了包括心脏搭桥、瓣膜置换、人工血管置换、先天性心脏病手术、心脏移植、经皮瓣膜手术、左心室辅助术等外科手术患者，提供共计92 615人次的外科住院康复，康复量较2022年提高了80%。门诊康复共计6138人次，较2022年提高0.5%。住院康复与门诊康复的数量较2019年分别提高3.4倍和2.5倍（图8-2）。

Cardiac rehabilitation Center expanded perioperative rehabilitation of cardiac surgery to 19 wards，including adult surgery ward，vascular surgery ward，structural ward，PICU，and SICU，intervening the patients who suffered surgeries，such as CABG，valve replacement，large vascular surgery，congenital heart surgery，heart transplantation，percutaneous valve surgery，left ventricular assist device surgery，etc. A total of 92，615 patients were treated for surgical inpatient rehabilitation，an increase of 80% over 2022. A total of 6，138 patients received outpatient rehabilitation，an increase of 0.5% over 2022. The number of inpatient rehabilitation and outpatient rehabilitation increased by 3.4 times and 2.5 times respectively compared with 2019（Figure 8-2）.

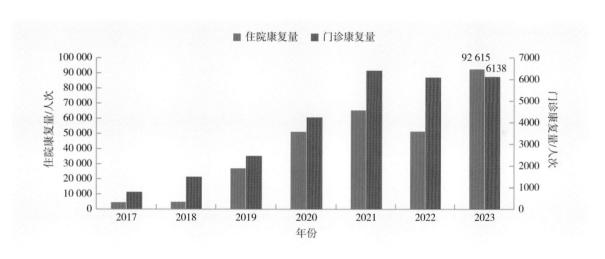

图8-2　2017—2023年心脏康复中心康复患者量

Figure 8-2　Volume of patients in cardiac rehabilitation centers in 2017—2023

2023年，心脏康复中心加大了对重症患者的康复力度，重视对于衰弱患者的筛查与干预，减少患者术前衰弱而引起的术后并发症，减少住院时间，提高患者生活质量。在挑战病情更重更难的患者同时，2023年中心继续保持以往的工作质量，全年接诊患者不良事件发生率0（图8-3）。

In 2023, Fuwai cardiac rehabilitation center strengthened the rehabilitation of severe patients, attached importance to the screening and intervention of frail patients, reduced postoperative complications caused by preoperative weakness, reduced hospitalization time and improved the quality of life of patients. While challenging more serious and difficult patients, in 2023, the center will continue to maintain the previous quality of work, and the incidence of adverse events of patients in the whole year was 0%（Figure 8-3）.

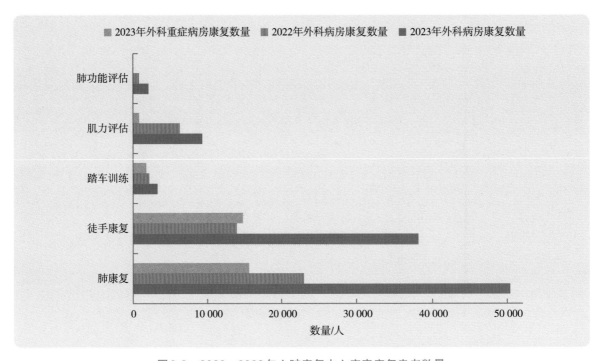

图8-3　2022—2023年心脏康复中心病房康复患者数量

Figure 8-3　Volume of patients in the cardiac rehabilitation center word in 2022—2023

心脏康复门诊进一步完善MDT团队综合干预患者康复的诊疗流程，及时评估患者存在的功能障碍，根据结果反馈积极开展治疗，提高患者就诊效率。并为患者提供居家康复方案，将治疗延续到出院后，促进患者长期保持健康的生活方式（图8-4）。

The cardiac rehabilitation clinic further improves the diagnosis and treatment process of MDT team's comprehensive intervention in patients' rehabilitation，timely evaluates patients' dysfunction，and actively carries out treatment according to the feedback of the results to improve the efficiency of patients' treatment. And provide patients with home rehabilitation programs to continue the treatment until after discharge and promote patients to maintain a healthy lifestyle for a long time（Figure 8-4）.

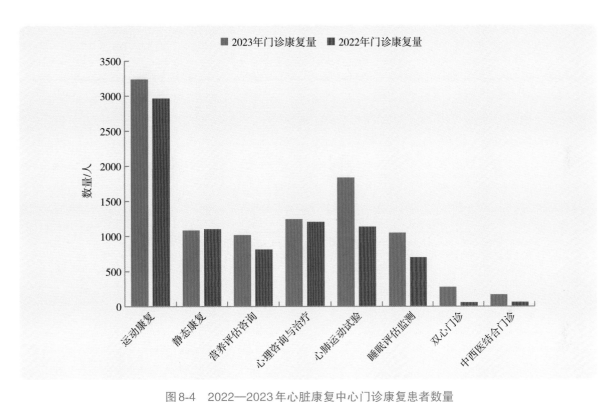

图8-4　2022—2023年心脏康复中心门诊康复患者数量

Figure 8-4　Volume of out-patients in the cardiac rehabilitation center in 2022—2023

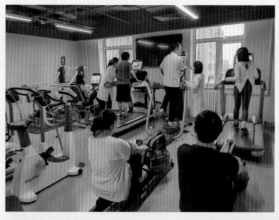
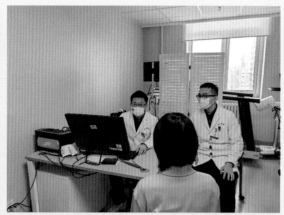
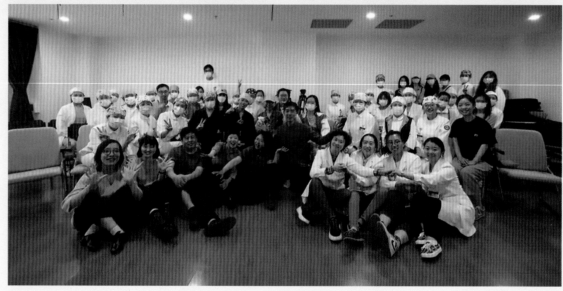

图8-5　特色心脏康复诊疗

Figure 8-5　Special cardiac rehabilitation

开展特色门诊

● 中西医结合门诊：通过传统中医手段（如太极、八段锦等传统运动和针灸、拔罐等），结合经典心脏康复治疗方式（如运动、营养等），为患者提供多元化的中西医结合的心脏康复干预方案。

● 双心门诊：由心理团队和心内科团队共同组成的双心门诊，服务心血管疾病合并精神心理障碍的患者。

● 在筛查心脏疾病的同时，可通过精神药物及心理咨询、生物反馈等非药物方式，对患者的精神心理问题进行同步诊疗。2023年共接诊双心诊疗患者276人。

● 2023年11月新开青少年群体双心诊疗，仅2个月接诊青少年患者102人次，为敏感期的青少年提供心理支持，鉴别心理或生理性的心脏不适。

● 晕厥患者双心诊疗：辅助晕厥患者的诊断，判断患者是否存在心因性的晕厥原因，纠正患者的焦虑情绪，缓解躯体化症状。

开展特殊人群的康复

● 对先天性心脏病患者进行心肺运动试验，为判断其心功能，评估生活质量提供依据，前后进行456人次的先心评估和随访。

● 对心脏移植和左心室辅助患者进行全周期康复。2023年共参与136名心脏移植/左心室辅助患者的康复，从入院开始干预患者，评估患者的衰弱，积极术前康复；术后从术后早期开始循序渐进的康复，直至患者出院。

● 随着阜外医院各个科室的建立，心脏康复中心逐步向综合康复中心发展。开展儿童先天性心脏病康复、周围神经病变康复、脊髓病变康复、脑血管病康复、骨关节康复等。

跨学科，多领域合作的创新康复项目

● 表达性艺术疗愈活动：共开展30期活动，通过有参与感的表达性艺术方式传达健康生活方式的重要性，激发对自身健康的关注，促进建立一个健康、智慧、自由、幸福的个体。

● 减脂训练营：以团体减脂的方式，以增肌减脂为目的，促进肥胖人群对健康体重的关注，满足不同需求人群，更加健康科学的降低体脂率。2023年共开展12期活动，参与者近150人。

special clinics:

● Integrated traditional Chinese and Western medicine clinic: through traditional Chinese medicine means（such as tai chi, Baduanjin and other traditional sports, acupuncture, cupping, etc.）, combined with classical cardiac rehabilitation treatment methods（such as exercise, nutrition, etc.）, to provide patients with a variety of integrated traditional Chinese and western medicine cardiac rehabilitation intervention programs.

● Cardio-Psychol clinic: the Cardio-Psychol clinic composed of a psychology team and a cardiology team, serving patients with cardiovascular disease and psychiatric disorders.

● At the same time of screening for heart disease, patients' mental and psychological problems can be simultaneously diagnosed and treated through psychotropic drugs, psychological counseling, biofeedback and other non-drug methods. In 2023, a total of 276 patients were admitted.

● In November, a new Cardio-Psychol clinic for teenagers was opened, and 102 patients were treated in just two months, providing psychological support for teenagers in sensitive period and distinguishing psychological or physiological heart discomfort.

● Cardio-psychol syncope clinic: assisting the diagnosis of syncope patients, judging whether there are psychological syncope causes, correcting patients' anxiety and relieving somatization symptoms.

for special people:

- Cardiopulmonary exercise test was carried out on patients with congenital heart disease, in order to provide basis for judging their cardiac function and evaluating their quality of life, and 456 people were evaluated and followed up。

- Full-cycle rehabilitation for patients with heart transplantation and left ventricular assist. In 2023, he participated in the rehabilitation of 136 patients with heart transplantation/ left ventricular assist, intervened patients from admission, evaluated patients' weakness and actively recovered before operation; After operation, the patient began to recover step by step from the early postoperative period until the patient was discharged from the hospital.

- With the establishment of various departments in Fuwai Hospital, the cardiac rehabilitation center has gradually developed into a comprehensive rehabilitation center. Carry out rehabilitation of children with congenital heart disease, peripheral neuropathy, myelopathy, cerebrovascular disease and muscle and joint rehabilitation.

Innovative rehabilitation projects with interdisciplinary and multi-field cooperation:

- Expressive art healing activities: A total of 30 activities were carried out to convey the importance of a healthy lifestyle through expressive art with a sense of participation, stimulate concern for one's own health and promote the establishment of a healthy, intelligent, free and happy individual.

- Weight-loss training camp: In the way of group fat-reducing, with the aim of gaining muscle and reducing fat, it promotes obese people to pay attention to healthy weight, and reduces body fat rate more healthily and scientifically. In 2023, 12 events were held with nearly 150 participants.

▶ 健康生活方式医学

创办品牌年会——中国健康生活方式医学大会（图8-6）。

Establish the annual meeting-China Healthy Lifestyle Medical Conference（Figure 8-6）.

2023年11月2—5日，举办第三届中国健康生活方式医学大会。总观看人数为261.9万，是首次举办生活方式医学沉浸式展览。

On November 2-5, 2023, the 3rd China Health Lifestyle Medicine Conference was held. The total number of visitors is 2.619 million, which is the first immersive exhibition of lifestyle medicine.

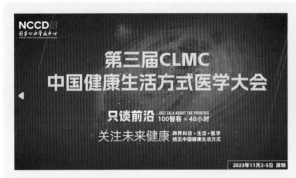 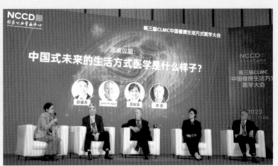

图8-6　中国健康生活方式医学大会

Figure 8-6　China Healthy Lifestyle Medical Conference

- 成立国家心血管病中心生活方式医学联盟（图8-7A）。
- Established the National Cardiovascular Center Lifestyle Medicine Alliance（Figure 8-7A）.

目前有93家单位加入，遍布全国二十余省及直辖市。

- 完成《生活方式医学》的译著（图8-7B）。
- Completed the translation of *Lifestyle Medicine*（Figure 8-7B）.

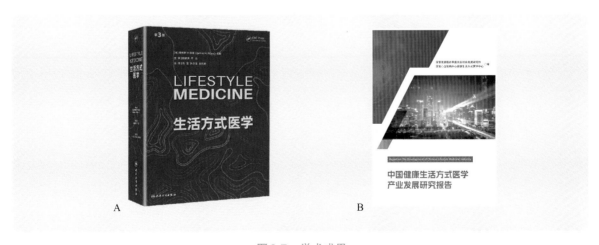

图8-7　学术成果

Figure 8-7　academic achievements

涵盖构建生活方式在临床医学各学科的全体系百科全书。

● 撰写中国健康生活方式医学产业发展研究报告（图8-7C）。

● Wrote a research report on the development of China's healthy lifestyle medical industry（Figure 8-7C）.

探究产业发展方向和趋势，提出壮大产业发展的相关政策建议。

● 发布《中国健康生活方式综合评价指数》。

● The Comprehensive Evaluation Index for Healthy Lifestyle in China has been released.

构建适合中国人群的健康生活方式的综合评价方法。

九、信息化、智能化助力医院高质量发展
Informatization and intelligence facilitates the advancement of high-quality healthcare in public hospitals

▶ **病历智能质控**

构建"自我识别、自动纠错、一键修改"的智能化病案管理"新模式"

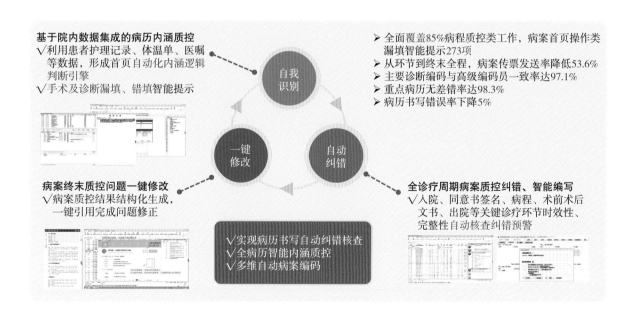

基于院内数据集成的病历内涵质控
√利用患者护理记录、体温单、医嘱等数据，形成首页自动化内涵逻辑判断引擎
√手术及诊断漏填、错填智能提示

病案终末质控问题一键修改
√病案质控结果结构化生成，一键引用完成问题修正

自我识别

一键修改

自动纠错

√实现病历书写自动纠错核查
√全病历智能内涵质控
√多维自动病案编码

➢ 全面覆盖85%病程质控类工作，病案首页操作类漏填智能提示273项
➢ 从环节到终末全程，病案传票发送率降低53.6%
➢ 主要诊断编码与高级编码员一致率达97.1%
➢ 重点病历无差错率达98.3%
➢ 病历书写错误率下降5%

全诊疗周期病案质控纠错、智能编写
√入院、同意书签名、病程、术前术后文书、出院等关键诊疗环节时效性、完整性自动核查纠错预警

▶ 智能抗生素管控

智能抗生素管理，PDCA知识反馈——外科抗生素合理使用监控

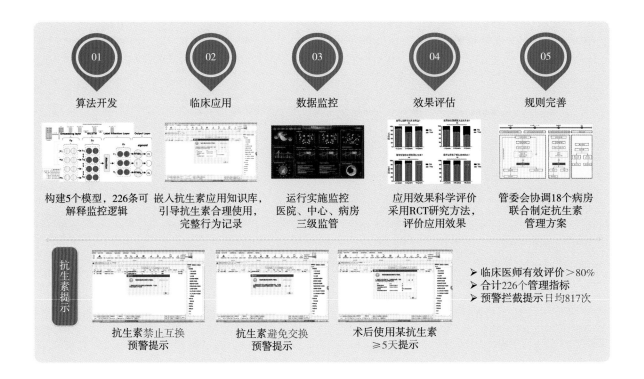

▶ 不良事件上报

利用客观数据和知识库，进行不良事件自动识别上报

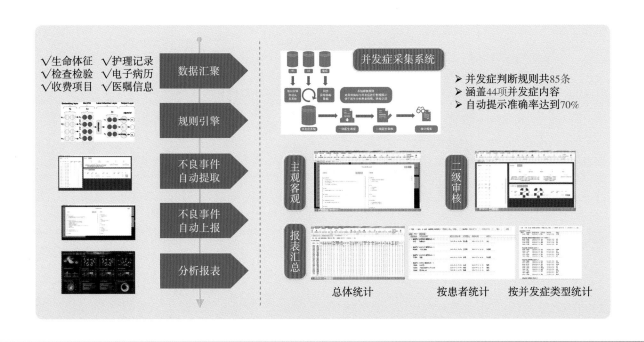

► 智能风险评估

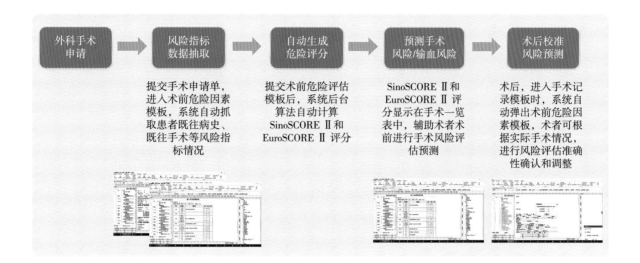

外科手术申请 → 风险指标数据抽取 → 自动生成危险评分 → 预测手术风险/输血风险 → 术后校准风险预测

提交手术申请单，进入术前危险因素模板，系统自动抓取患者既往病史、既往手术等风险指标情况

提交术前危险评估模板后，系统后台算法自动计算SinoSCORE II 和 EuroSCORE II 评分

SinoSCORE II 和 EuroSCORE II 评分显示在手术一览表中，辅助术者术前进行手术风险评估预测

术后，进入手术记录模板时，系统自动弹出术前危险因素模板，术者可根据实际手术情况，进行风险评估准确性确认和调整

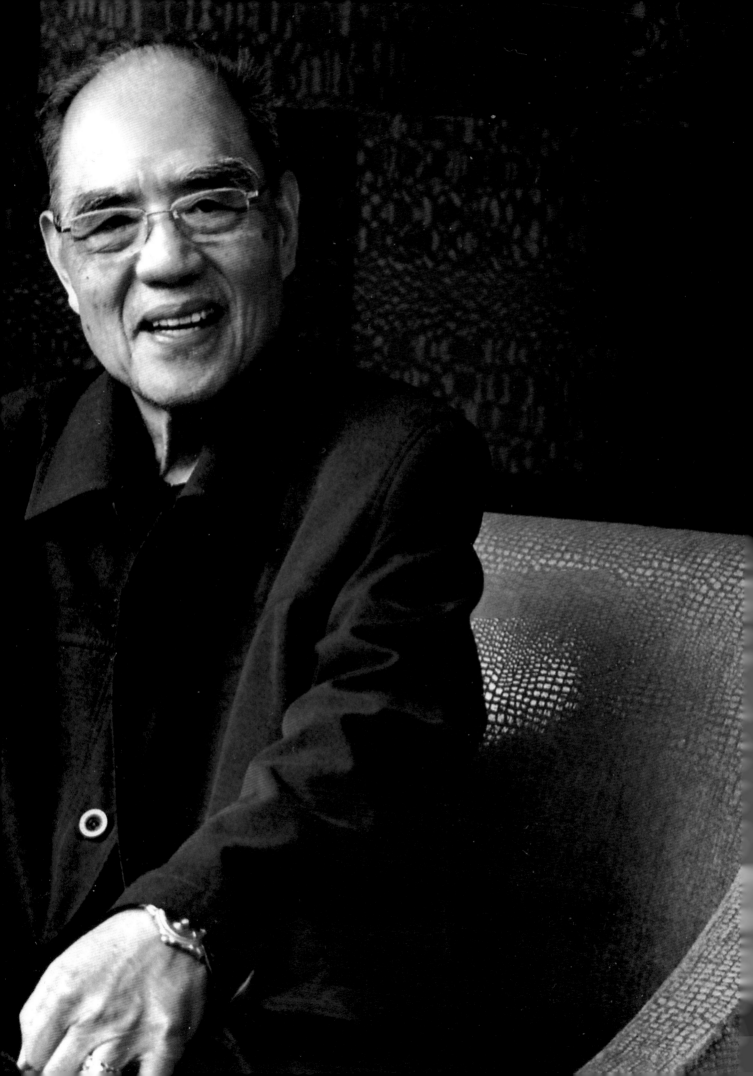

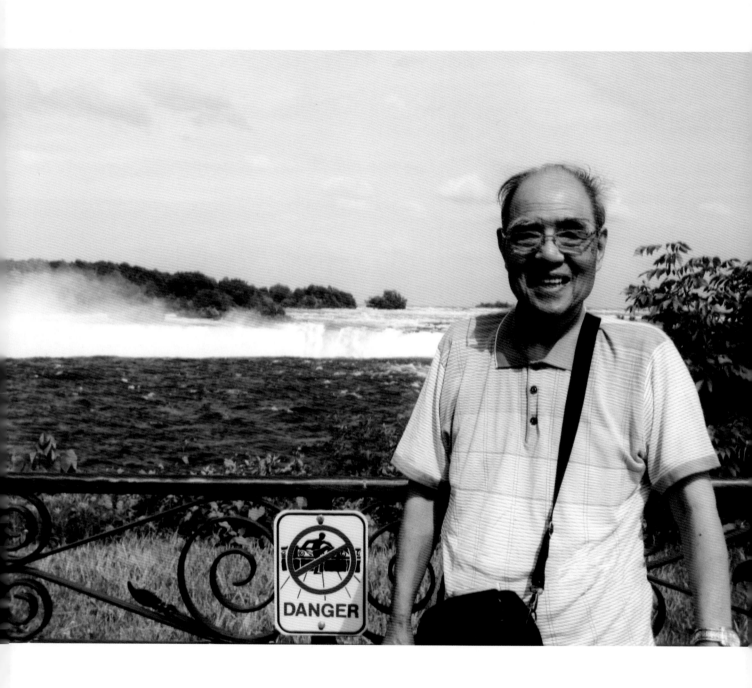